Natural Beauty Alchemy

Natural Beauty Alchemy

Make Your Own Organic Cleansers, Creams, Serums, Shampoos, Balms, and More

FIFI M. MAACARON

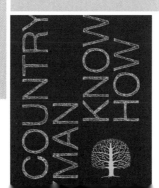

COUNTRYMAN KNOW HOW

Published by
THE COUNTRYMAN PRESS
P.O. Box 748, Woodstock, VT 05091

Distributed by
W. W. NORTON & COMPANY, INC
500 Fifth Avenue, New York, NY 10110

Printed in the United States

Natural Beauty Alchemy
978-1-58157-272-8

10 9 8 7 6 5 4 3 2 1

AN IDEA REMAINS AN IDEA,
UNTIL IT IS CRAFTED WITH PASSION!

Through the challenges, with a lot of time, effort,
and determination, this project came together.

For my family, who supported and motivated me when I needed it
most; for my beautiful mother, who did everything only a mother can
do; for my friends, who were amazing first enthusiasts; and for every
natural beauty believer, a heartfelt thank you.

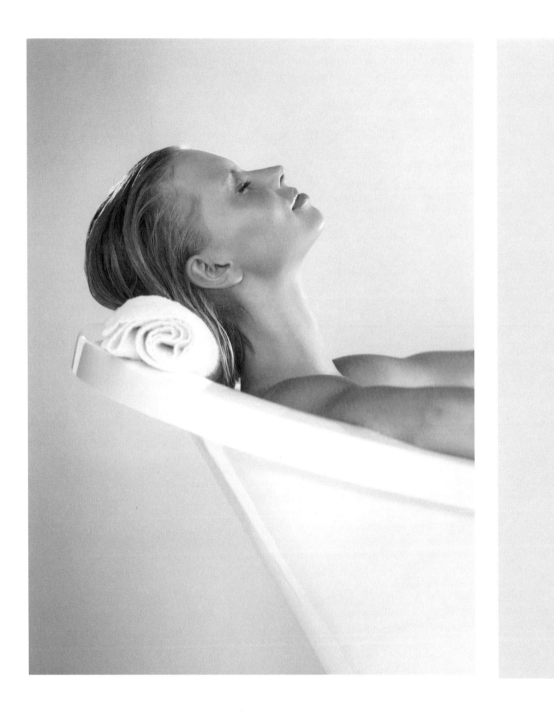

CONTENTS

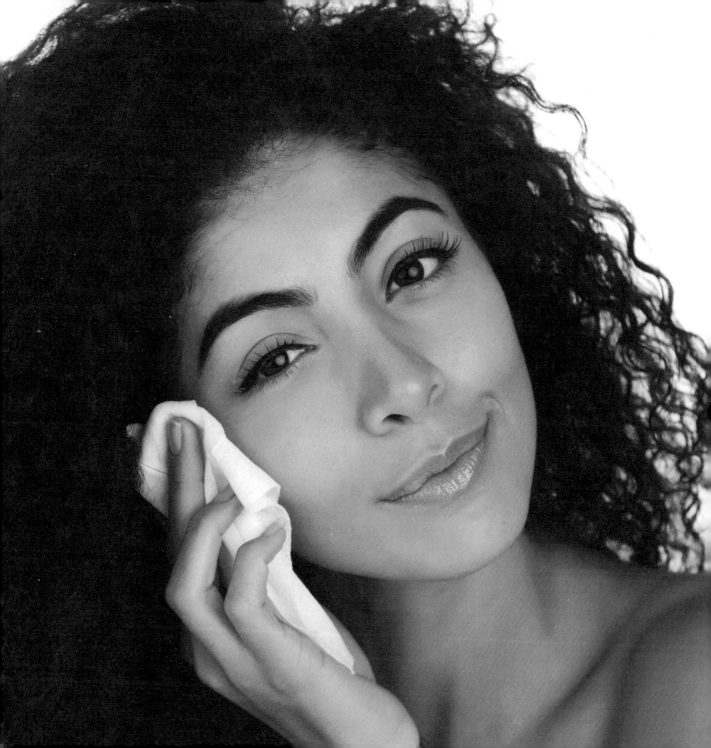

What Is Beauty?

Beauty is a perceptual concept that grows with individuals of every society and culture.

As we begin to understand what it means and grasp its dimensions, we learn to appreciate it and search for it in every facet of our lives. We also attempt to bring beauty into our daily lives by incorporating beautiful things into our surrounding environment and by trying to beautify our own appearance.

Most women, men, and children have an innate desire to look and feel beautiful inside and out, and there is a certain harmony that often links inner and outer beauty and reflects the result to the outside.

Each person defines and implements beauty in a different way, but despite the subjectivity, a huge platform remains common ground for most people in search of a more "beautiful" look. That platform is nothing but the vast field of cosmetics.

Making cosmetics has always been part of human history, and recipes are part of popular tradi-tions and folklores, preserved on papyri and cher-ished by descendants for generations.

Very simple and basic, most preparations were concocted from naturally available and locally grown ingredients: Cleopatra bathed in milk and honey; Romans used olive oil and rose water to make creams; Arabs made perfumes from agarwood (called *oud*), amber, and saffron.

As humanity evolved, the complexity of cosmet-ics evolved, as well. It became possible to transition from old-world beauty traditions to new age formu-las, and modern techniques allowed packing some beauty goodness into jars and tubes of all shapes and colors.

Newer technologies and emerging scientific pro-tocols endorsed the benefits of countless ingredients. Herbal extracts have been purified and standardized;

active molecules have been identified, analyzed, and documented; and placebo controlled clinical trials have been conducted to test efficacy claims.

Such an abundance of scientific information made it possible to concretely understand the secrets to the success of various formulations, to appreciate numerous natural ingredients, to choose what is most suitable for every specific need and use it in an optimal way for optimum results.

Cosmetics concretized modern alchemy and managed to pour some of the utopic beauty fountain into individual jars that require only simple steps to nurture, soothe, protect, and rejuvenate skin.

Even though this may sound a little like a fairytale, it is far from being one. What was once folklore heritage has become the high-profit industry of the fifty-billion-dollar U.S. cosmetics empire. With countless chemical innovations and high-tech industrialization, the fast-paced world of cosmetics has grown further and further apart from its natural sources and acquired an unpleasantly dense chemical complexity, with a predominant emphasis on efficacy and little focus on safety and tolerability. With the quasi absence of official regulations, manufacturers began comfortably including an increasing number of questionable ingredients for profitability reasons such as extending shelf life and reducing costs.

For that reason, for many, cosmetics themselves needed a makeover.

Several public interest groups such as professional authors, feminists, animal rights activists, environmentalists, and many others campaign against this humongous empire of cosmetics and broadcast data to raise awareness at the consumer level.

Consumers, mostly women, understand that what makes them look prettier may not be good for them. They realize that there may be ugly harsh ingredients inside their beauty products; that what is offered as a solution to a need may not be what they want or how they want it; that unfortunately, unethical, profit-driven marketing exists and they do not want to be misled.

More exigent consumers divorced glamorous brands and started a search for safer, better-tolerated, time-tested, more natural and skin-friendly solutions in an attempt to build their own independent, effective, transparent, and honest beauty regimens.

While manufacturers still try to drive market demand toward their own products through various strategies, such as TV commercials, price drops or coupons, and attractive packaging, other decision factors are affecting choices, making it obvious to conventional product manufacturers that there has been a considerable shift in purchasing behavior, with fewer impulsive and more informed consumers. Those emerging market dynamics forced the creation of a new, more natural category of cosmetics that targets the lost customers, avoiding questionable ingredients and including more naturally sourced, skin-friendly components.

Even though those changes have been welcomed, problems have not been completely solved, and the new products have created a new labyrinth. Poor regulations and vague standardization guidelines have led many consumers to wonder why finding the right products to upgrade their beauty arsenal has become so difficult, complicated by stretched claims, countless different logos, and lengthy lists of ingredients that often include incoherent information and require expert analysis. Thus, the decision to shift to more natural skin care hasn't always translated to easily finding satisfactory products according to "natural" criteria.

As a consequence, a vast multitude of skin care product users pressed the "reset" button of their beauty routines, and many others are about to do the same; all of them are in need of unbiased, trustworthy information, as well as better alternatives.

Natural Beauty Alchemy will decode the secrets of the trade and dissipate the mystery surrounding the world of cosmetics. The professional-level information, up-to-date research, and impartial opinions in this book will help you to understand the dynamics behind the fascinating world of skin care. Ingredients are analyzed, benefits are listed, technicalities are explained in detail, and every bit of knowledge is presented in such a way that readers can understand.

Every woman will be able to take charge of her own beauty regimen, understand what her skin needs, and provide it with the best care without compromise.

You will be able to understand skin, skin care, and cosmetics and interpret ingredients as individual components that build the entity and the identity of a product. You will know what each ingredient is, its role within a formula, how natural it is, and what benefits it can bring. You will appreciate the practical meaning of existing certifications and what they stand for in regard to ingredients, as well as to finished products. You will be able to analyze formulas and evaluate components, authenticity, coherence, and expected benefits.

This book will prepare you to choose a wide array of products that will cater to all your beauty needs in a customized, natural, trustworthy way. A generous, broad, and authentic collection of one hundred formulas inspired from different parts of the world will cover all skin care needs, making beauty rituals more authentic and more pleasurable.

Built on solid scientific standards, the information in this book provides a logical and fun way of making your own beauty products according to precise formulations that are safe, easy, and effective.

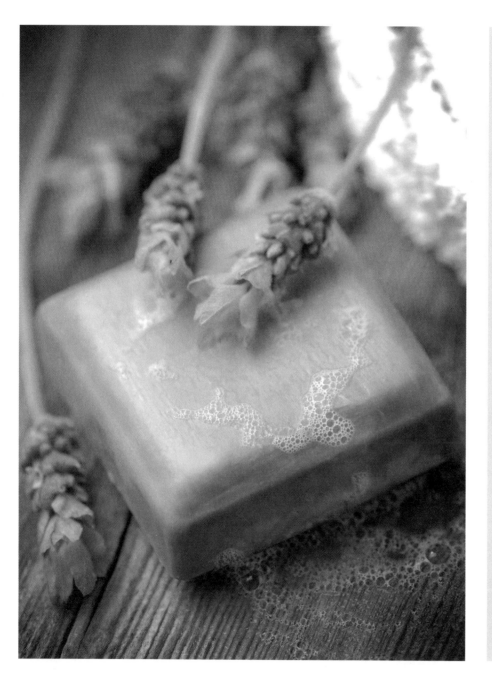

Understanding Natural Skin Care and Ingredients

1

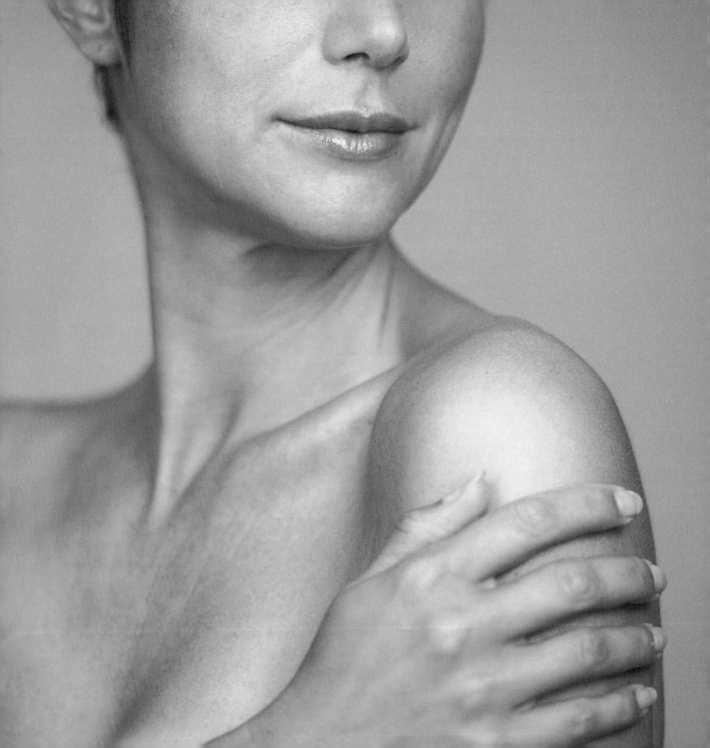

Skin

Definition, Role, and Structure

Skin is the exterior organ that covers the human body, as well as the body of other vertebrates. It is the first layer that comes in contact with exterior factors, helping to protect us from external dangers. Because of its dense network of sensitive nerve endings, skin acts as a sensory organ as well. It also helps regulate our body temperature and is capable of activating vitamin D after UV exposure.

Skin thickness varies greatly across the human body; it is thinnest around the eyes, where wrinkles tend to first appear, while the heels and palms are covered with notably denser skin.

It was long believed that skin was an impermeable barrier. Although it is true that skin does not allow bigger compounds to penetrate it, such belief was revised after the skin was found to be permeable to many substances, including most skin care products. This permeability can allow the introduction of chemicals (such as coal tar and phthalates) into the human body. The skin can also be a targeted port of entry for numerous drugs, whose active ingredients (such as hormones or nitroglycerin) are delivered to the circulatory system, via the skin, through medicated creams, ointments, or patches.

The skin is divided into three layers:

1. epidermis (the most exterior)

2. dermis

3. hypodermis

The epidermis is further divided into strata or layers: stratum corneum (the most exterior),

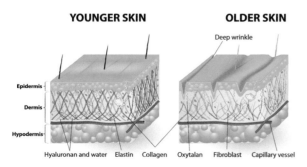

YOUNGER SKIN — OLDER SKIN

Epidermis · Dermis · Hypodermis

Deep wrinkle

Hyaluronan and water · Elastin · Collagen · Oxytalan · Fibroblast · Capillary vessel

stratum granulosum, stratum spinosum, and stratum germinativum.

Keratinocytes, which make up to 95 percent of the epidermis cells, migrate from the stratum germinativum up toward the stratum corneum. As this migration occurs, keratinocytes become highly organized, secrete keratin (the main protein of the epidermis) and lipids, lose their nuclei (become dead cells), and are then shed through the natural process of desquamation, or peeling.

The epidermis and dermis meet at the level of the basement membrane, which is a thin layer of fibers. The dermis is a dense network of connective tissues, blood and lymphatic vessels, nerve endings, hair follicles, and sweat and sebaceous glands. The hypodermis is a connective tissue that ties the dermis to the muscles, bones, vessels, and nerves. It hosts adipose cells (fat cells), collagen cells, and sweat glands. A reduction in the mass of this section of the skin contributes to skin sagging.

Moisturizers can significantly hydrate only the upper layers of the epidermis. Actual nutrition of deeper epidermis cells happens by diffusion from a network of capillaries found in the underlying dermis, which is why proper hydration and balanced nutrition are strong contributors to better-looking skin.

Unlike moisturizers, which act at the level of the upper layers of the epidermis, pharmaceutical topical drugs are formulated to achieve deeper skin penetration. The active ingredient is delivered to deeper layers, where it can exert a local or systemic effect.

Examples of such drugs include the nitroglycerin patch, anti-inflammatory creams, and medicated gels.

Skin care products can also be formulated with a deeper penetration objective; for example, a product designed to improve collagen production might need to incorporate penetration enhancers into the formula to maximize the delivery of its collagen-promoting ingredients. Such formulas can be micro-emulsions, whose bipolar droplet size encourages passage through skin layers; or they can contain powerful solvents which will transport other ingredients to lower skin levels. Such formulations may not totally comply with the FDA's definition of cosmetics, which are not supposed to affect bodily functions; but they remain popular because of the promised results.

Skin Types

There are five basic skin types: normal, oily, dry, combination, and sensitive.

Normal skin has an adequate balance of sebum and moisture, which contributes to its smooth and even surface. Normal skin does not feel greasy or dry, has good elasticity, and tolerates most environmental challenges. It needs only basic care and rarely requires special treatment regimens.

Oily skin has mild to moderately overactive sebaceous glands, which lead to an excess in sebum production. Skin feels greasy to the touch, especially on the nose and forehead areas, and requires daily or twice daily cleaning to remove accumulated oils. Excess sebum can gather both dust and bacteria, which is why oily skin is prone to black and white heads, as well as blemishes and acne. Astringents are widely used on oily skin, since they decrease the size of pores and help reduce sebum production. Antibacterial agents are also useful in controlling bacterial proliferation. Nevertheless, excess cleaning is not recommended because it is thought to further stimulate sebaceous glands and contribute to maximized sebum production and a significant rebound effect, especially when care is withheld.

Dry skin lacks both oily secretions and moisture. Because of the insufficient quantity of sebum produced by the sebaceous glands, the skin's coating is unable to adequately prevent moisture loss and maintain a well-hydrated skin. Dry skin tends to wrinkle more easily and can become chapped in challenging weather conditions such as extreme cold. It is very important to apply moisturizers and creams specially formulated for dry skin, which tolerates higher percentages of oils, or even butters.

Combination skin, a very common type of skin, is a mixture of both dry and oily skin, in which oily skin covers the forehead, nose, and chin (the T-zone), and dry skin covers the cheeks and the area around the eyes. Theoretically, each zone should be treated according to its type, unless the skin care regimen is specifically designed for combination skin.

Sensitive skin often has a very fine texture and poor tolerance to many elements, which can turn out to be irritating and sensitizing. Such elements could be soap, synthetic fragrances, artificial preservatives, dyes, and even temperature changes and aggressive weather. Simple, fragrance-free, hypoallergenic, and purely natural skin care products are usually the best regimens for sensitive skin types.

Skin Patch Test

Because skin reactions can be unpredictable, testing the skin's tolerance to a new product is essential to detect potential allergies. This is usually done prior to using any product for the first time, whether it is store-bought or homemade. It is very easy to test your skin for a reaction prior to normal application by applying a little of the product on a small and discreet area; it takes only twenty-four hours to get results. Homemade formulations are usually very well tolerated; most reactions tend to occur when acidic compounds (such as lemon juice or yogurt) are included. The formulas in this book are designed to include well-tolerated amounts of such ingredients, so that they can be effective while reducing the risk of sensitivity.

People with sensitive skin and people who tend to break out easily should be more cautious when trying new products. Still, because every person's skin is unique, and because tolerability varies greatly between individuals, a skin patch test is highly advisable, no matter the skin type, to avoid potential skin reactions.

Apply a pea-size amount of the product to the inside of your elbow. Cover with gauze and wait for twenty-four hours before removing it. Covering the test area with gauze prevents the product from being rubbed off. Avoid getting the bandage wet during testing time. Remove the patch immediately if you notice any signs of allergy such as redness, swelling, rash, itching, or tingling or burning sensations. If this happens, rinse the affected skin area with plenty of warm water, without scrubbing to avoid further irritation, and discontinue the product's use. Contact a dermatologist if your symptoms do not improve. Otherwise, remove the gauze after twenty-four hours and examine the area for any signs of allergy. No reaction means that it should be okay to use the product. Discontinue use if a reaction occurs upon secondary applications.

Skin Nutrients

Multiple components come together to form and maintain skin. Water, proteins, fats, minerals, vitamins, and other nutrients are essential for maintaining the balance of skin and mucosal tissues. Skin is capable of renewing itself every twenty-seven days, on average. Older cells are lost through shedding, and newly differentiated ones replace them. Diet and skin care have a great effect on skin cells, since skin needs specific nutrients that can be provided through diet, topically, or both. Studies have shown that diets rich in vegetables, fruits, fish, and olive oil contribute to better-looking skin. It is also established that adequate hydration can lead to better skin moisture levels.

PROTEINS AND AMINO ACIDS

Proteins are an important component of skin cells, with the two most prevalent ones being collagen and keratin. While collagen alone accounts for 75 percent of skin, keratin is mostly present in the epidermis and is the main component of hair and nails. Collagen and elastin, another protein, are mainly part of the dermis, where both proteins are in charge of maintaining adequate skin elasticity and support. It is within the dermis that wrinkles form.

Adequate supplementation of proteins, whether sourced from animals or vegetables, is essential for maintaining healthy skin and for allowing wounds to heal. Quality proteins and amino acids such as lysine, proline, arginine, and glycine are important for skin maintenance and collagen health and can be found in a variety of dietary sources, including peanuts, walnuts, flaxseeds, chickpeas, quinoa, dairy, egg whites, fish, and poultry.

It is also important to maintain sufficient levels of vitamin C, since it is a co-player involved in in-vivo amino acid production (hydroxyproline). Additionally, it is a valuable antioxidant that plays an important role in preserving collagen and preventing its breakdown.

UNSATURATED FATTY ACIDS

Unsaturated fatty acids are so called because they possess one or more double bonds in their carbon main chain molecule. Monounsaturated fatty acids have a single double bond between the main chain carbon atoms; polyunsaturated fatty acids have multiple double bonds between the main chain carbon atoms. Polyunsaturated fatty acids (PUFA), or essen-

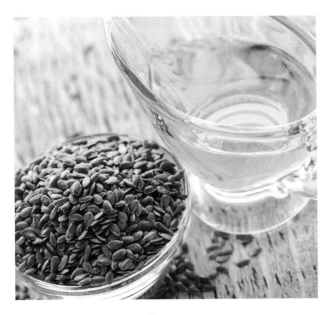

tial fatty acids, are of great importance to the skin. Vegetable oils are rich in essential fatty acids.

Essential fatty acids are acids that the human body needs but is unable to synthesize or produce—such as linoleic acid (LA) and alpha linolenic acid (ALA). They are therefore necessary as part of the diet.

Polyunsaturated acids are divided into the following types:

1. Omega-3 polyunsaturated fatty acids: These are named as such because the first double bond occurs between the third and fourth carbon atom from the omega end of the chain. They are abundant in fish such as sardines, mackerel, salmon, scallops, and halibut, as well as in flaxseeds and walnuts. They are present to a lesser extent in many other sources, such as olive oil, beans, and tofu. Specific omega-3s of physiological importance to human beings are ALA (alpha linolenic acid), DHA (docosahexaenoic acid), and EPA (eicosapentaenoic acid). The human body can produce, to some extent, DHA and EPA from ALA, but not at the skin level, where the appropriate enzymes are absent. That is why they are considered essential fatty acids. Flaxseed oil (also known as linseed oil) and walnut oil are both high in ALA.

2. Omega-6 polyunsaturated acids: These are named as such because the first double bond occurs after the sixth carbon atom from the omega end of the chain. Omega-6s include GLA (gamma linolenic acid), DGLA (dihomo GLA), AA (arachidonic acid), and LA (linoleic acid). The human body can produce GLA and AA from LA, but, again, not at the skin level, where the appropriate enzymes are absent. Evening primrose and borage oils are high in GLA. Sunflower and safflower oils are rich in LA.

3. Omega-9 polyunsaturated acids: These are named as such because the first double bond occurs after the ninth carbon atom from the omega end of the main chain; examples include oleic acid, eicosenoic acid, and others.

4. There are also conjugated fatty acids and other polyunsaturates that are not considered essential fatty acids.

Omega-6 essential fatty acids are considered skin building blocks and are incorporated into ceramides, a type of lipid molecule; omega-3s are anti-inflammatory and protect skin from sun damage.

It is established now that essential fatty acids are important for many metabolic functions of the body. Individual levels of these, as well as their relative proportions, may have significant physiological impact. Research shows that western diets are often too elevated in omega-6 oils and relatively low in omega-3s, with unhealthy ratios, exceeding by multiple times the recommended omega-6 to omega-3 ratio of between 1:1 and 4:1.

VITAMINS AND MINERALS

Vitamins and minerals are valuable micronutrients, essential for optimal bodily functions. A number of those micronutrients are specifically important for skin cell maintenance.

Vitamin A

Vitamin A and its precursors, also known as retinoids, are vital for skin health. Animal sources (such as liver and eggs) provide retinol precursors. Retinol itself is then converted to retinoic acid, which contributes to rejuvenating skin by acting as a growth factor for epithelial cells.

Vegetable sources (such as carrots and spinach) provide another kind of pro-vitamin A, which are pigments known as carotenoids. In humans, four different types of carotenoids are able to exhibit vitamin A activity: alpha-carotene, beta-carotene, gamma-carotene, and beta-cryptoxanthin.

Vitamin A is essential for the adequate functioning of epithelial cells, and its deficiency can lead to the replacement of "mucus-secreting cells" by "keratin-producing cells," which can result in severely dry skin (known as *xerosis*). Vitamin A is also an important antioxidant that plays an essential role in maintaining vision and eye health.

Retinyl palmitate, which is a vitamin A precursor, is widely used in topical creams. It is ultimately converted to retinoic acid, an active form of vitamin A. Tretinoin (also known as ATRA: all-trans retinoic acid) is used to treat skin conditions such as acne and follicular keratosis.

Isotretinoin is reserved for cystic acne, because it can effectively counteract sebaceous glands. Since it could cause fetal harm, its use has strict medical restrictions.

Excessive intake of vitamin A or its derivatives can result in toxicity, which is why it is advisable not to exceed the recommended daily dose. Also, pregnant women and women who intend to or might become pregnant should consult with their physician regarding vitamin A and carotenoid intake (including topical applications) due to the risk of fetal harm related to high vitamin A levels.

Vitamin E

Also known as tocopherol and tocotrienol, vitamin E plays various physiological roles and is particularly

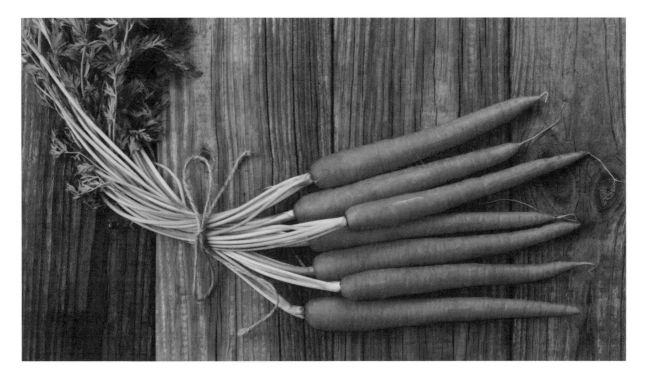

important for the skin. Because it is a natural antioxidant, it is capable of protecting skin cells from free radicals and preventing skin aging. It reduces sunspots and wrinkles and is also beneficial in cases of psoriasis and erythema.

Vitamin E is widely added to skin care formulations, including sun care products, since it helps improve the efficacy of sunscreens. It is also widely used as a preservative in food and skin care products, where it protects oils from oxidation and helps extend shelf life.

Vegetable oils and nuts are excellent dietary sources of vitamin E. Low-fat diets can result in a low intake of vitamin E unless fortified sources are included. However, excessive intake of vitamin E may increase the risk of bleeding; people with certain medical conditions should consult with their physician prior to supplementing with vitamin E.

Vitamin B5

Also known as pantothenic acid, vitamin B5 is part of the vitamin B complex. It acts as a skin moisturizer and hydrator and is capable of improving skin elasticity and softness. Studies have shown that it can help in skin regeneration. It can also counteract hair loss and is beneficial for hair and nail health.

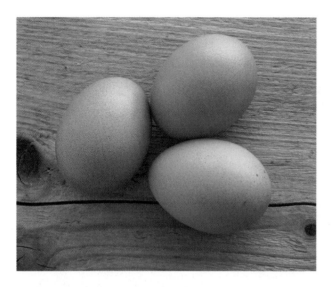

Meat, vegetables, grains, legumes, eggs, and milk are good sources of vitamin B5.

Vitamin C

Sometimes known as ascorbic acid, Vitamin C is a powerful antioxidant. It is essential for skin because it plays a key role in collagen synthesis. Present in both the epidermis and the dermis, vitamin C acts against damaging free radicals and slows collagen breakdown, wrinkle formation, skin aging, age spots, and sun damage. It is also capable of recycling vitamin E by reversing its oxidation.

Foods rich in vitamin C include oranges, grapefruits, parsley, broccoli, strawberries, and potatoes.

Topically, vitamin C is used to reverse skin aging, improve the appearance of sunspots, and prevent wrinkle formation.

Copper

Copper is a valuable trace mineral that plays major important roles in the body. It is essential for the adequate activity of the antioxidant enzyme *super oxide dismutase* and regulates the activity of *lysyl oxidase*, an enzyme needed for collagen formation in bones, connective tissues, and skin. Copper is also essential for melanin production.

The best sources of copper are liver, oysters, tahini, sesame seeds, cashews and other nuts, squid, and lobster.

Manganese

Manganese is a heavy metal needed in trace amounts for multiple bodily functions. It plays a structural role in skin collagen synthesis. It also activates an enzyme called prolidase, which is responsible for providing proline, an amino acid that is incorporated into collagen during its synthesis.

Whole grains, nuts, and leafy vegetables are good food sources of manganese.

Silica

Silica plays a role in preserving skin elasticity.

The best food sources for silica include leeks, green beans, garbanzo beans, strawberries, cucumber, mango, celery, and asparagus.

Zinc

Zinc is an essential mineral that has antioxidant properties and plays key physiological roles. Zinc deficiency has been linked to acne, since zinc helps regulate sebum production and tame hormones associated with acne.

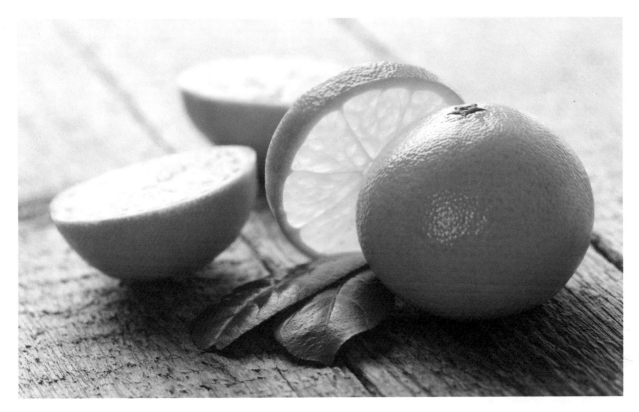

Oysters, pumpkin seeds and nuts, ginger, oats, and eggs are excellent sources of zinc.

Antioxidants

Antioxidants are essential in fighting harmful free radicals and protecting cellular DNA. They are abundant in fruits such as berries and apples, vegetables such as broccoli and tomatoes, nuts and seeds, and various spices.

Vitamins A, C, and E are known antioxidants. Oil-soluble vitamin E is present in many vegetable oils and protects the oils from rancidity and oxidation of double bonds.

Many vegetable oils are capable of providing a number of additional antioxidants that help protect skin from sun damage, premature aging, and collagen breakage. Antioxidants including beta-carotene, lycopene, lutein, xanthin, phytosterols, flavonoids, and polyphenols can be found in many vegetable oils, depending on the source of that oil.

Vegetable oils that are rich in antioxidants include blueberry seed oil, pomegranate seed oil, tomato seed oil, and walnut oil, among others.

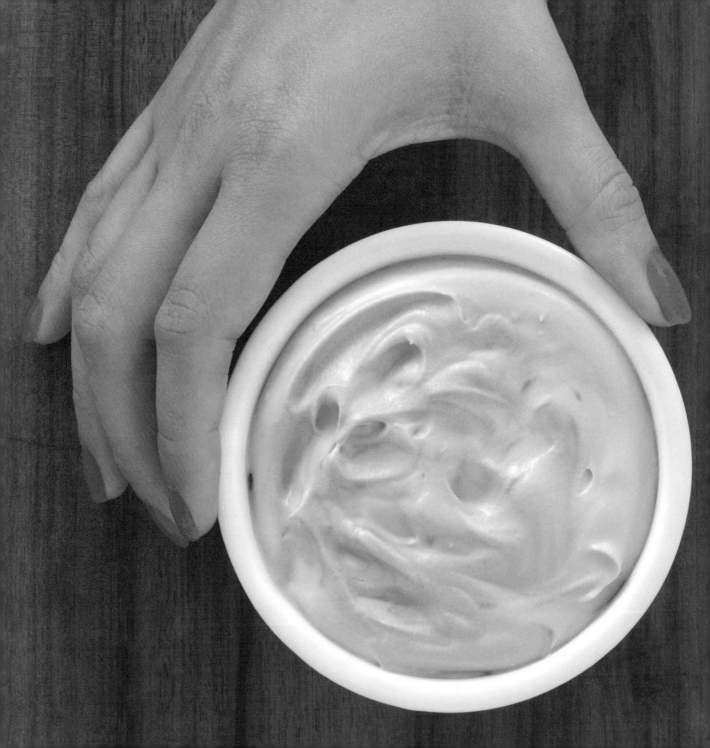

CHAPTER 2

Skin Care Categories

Two categories of products join each other under the vast umbrella of so-called cosmetics: makeup and skin care products. While makeup includes products such as lipsticks, foundation, mascara, eye shadow, and blush, skin care products include lotions and creams, sunscreens, facial serums, massage or tanning oils, baby skin care products, facial masks, scrubs, hand sanitizers, and many others.

Although lotions and creams are the most prevalent forms of skin care products, there are many other less ubiquitous formulations such as solutions, suspensions, gels, oils, ointments, balms, and even powders.

Lotions and Creams

Lotions and creams are emulsions formed by dispersion of an oil phase into an aqueous phase or an aqueous phase into an oil phase. The emulsion is then called an oil-in-water or water-in-oil emulsion, respectively. Generally speaking, most lotions are oil-in-water because they are more pleasant to the touch and do not leave a greasy residue. Because of the immiscibility of the two phases, oil droplets are dispersed and stabilized within the continuous aqueous phase with the aid of an emulsifier, which can also act as a surfactant—as in, for example, lecithin and cetearyl alcohol. Sometimes a thickener, such as gum or starch, is also used to bring more stability to the emulsion by increasing the viscosity of the continuous phase and reducing the risk of separation of the two phases.

Lotions, which are thinner than creams, are usually reserved for body formulations since they are easier to spread.

Solutions

Solutions are liquid formulations made of soluble solids dissolved in an aqueous phase and, perhaps, other water-miscible liquids, such as rubbing alcohol. Because of their high water content, and if they do not contain enough rubbing alcohol, solutions may need preservatives.

Suspensions

Suspensions are made of insoluble solid particles that remain suspended within the continuous phase. Although some settling might occur, the suspension can be recovered by shaking the container prior to application. Caking is a more serious issue, because it is more difficult to reverse than settling.

Examples of suspensions include bead or clay-based exfoliators.

Gels

Gels are semisolid solutions or suspensions in which the water phase is thickened and transformed into a homogenous gel. Gels are more stable than liquid suspensions because settling is less likely to occur. Gelling agents include gums and cellulose derivatives. Gels are refreshing and have a pleasant cosmetic feel due to the high water content, without greasy residue.

Examples of gels include hand sanitizers.

Oils

Oils are very simple to make because they are a mixture of miscible components and so, unlike solutions, do not require preservation. The absence of water makes oily preparations less favorable for bacterial growth. As for the oxidation that might occur within the oils, unsaturated fatty acids, it can be slowed down by adding antioxidants such as vitamin E and by storing the final preparation in an amber bottle, away from light and heat, which may act as oxidation catalyzers. Therapeutic active oils or fragrant essential oils are often diluted with neutral or carrier oils to bring their concentration to adequate levels.

Oils are mainly preferred for dry skin as facial serums, for hair care, and for body massages.

Ointments

Ointments are highly viscous formulations made mostly of thick bases such as lanolin, with oils and oil-miscible ingredients. There is little to no water content in ointments. They are very greasy and have poor cosmetic appeal.

Ointments are much more common in the pharmaceutical field, examples including corticosteroids and antibiotic ointments.

Balms

Balms are solidified ointments; they include a high proportion of waxes and butters, which solidify at room temperature. Balms are very easy to make and require no preservatives. They are favored when

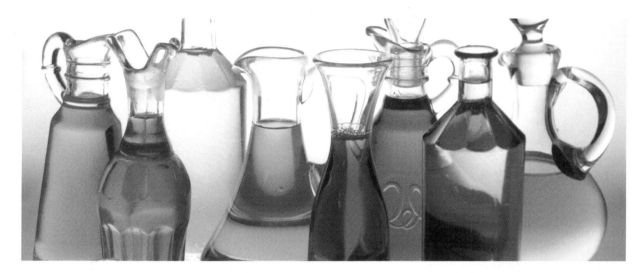

an occlusive effect is needed, such as when skin is severely damaged by aggressive weather.

Examples include lip and heel balms.

Powders

Cosmetic powders are fine, solid powders that can be offered loose or compacted, often blended with coloring pigments and possibly other agents to improve fluidity, prevent caking, or bring some benefits to the skin.

Examples include mineral and baby powder.

Ice Cubes, Steam Baths, and Warm Compresses

Ice cubes, steam baths, and warm compresses are considered concoctions rather than real skin care preparations and are often used for various skin ailments.

There is a common belief that applying cold (ice cubes or refrigerated moisturizers) to the skin helps firm and tighten it. Such "tightening" of the skin is temporary, however, and cold will constrict the blood vessels and thus decrease immediate absorption of the applied "nutrients."

Steam baths are a common practice to open pores and facilitate skin cleaning and blackhead removal. Steam can be generated by hot water with or without additives. This practice is not recommended for people with certain medical conditions, including asthma, COPD, and cardiovascular disease, or for pregnant women.

Cold or warm compresses and poultices are often applied to swollen areas such as puffy eyelids. It is important that the temperature of the compress respects the skin's tolerance. People with rosacea or dilated blood vessels should check with their dermatologist before using compresses or poultices.

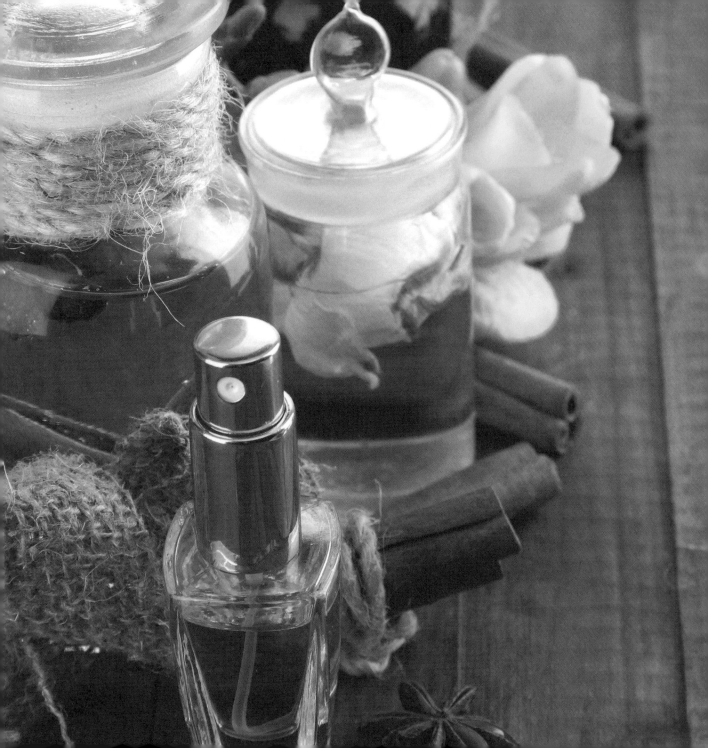

CHAPTER 3

Ingredients

An increasing number of ingredients are used in skin care formulations, both natural or organic and conventional. Water, hydrosols, oils, butters, waxes, emulsifiers, thickeners, preservatives, fragrances, essential oils, colors, pigments, herbal extracts, vitamins, minerals, peptides, rubbing alcohol, and many others are omnipresent in many skin care products. Knowing more about those ingredients—what they are, why they are part of the formula, what benefits they bring, and how they should be used— will help every beauty enthusiast to understand a beauty product formulation and make informed and customized choices. A list of possible substitutions can be found on page 260.

Understanding the ingredients is also a mandatory step prior to making your own cosmetics. Adequate knowledge will help you analyze formulas and make wise substitutions and potential adjustments to the recipe.

Water

Water is often the first ingredient in the formulation of skin care products. It constitutes the greatest percentage of the ingredients in facial creams and lotions, an average of 60 percent.

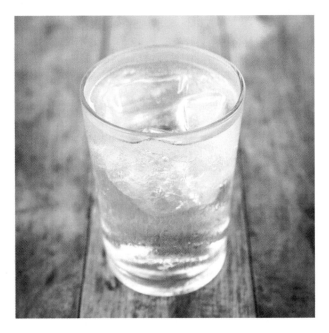

The quality of water that is incorporated into a cosmetic is monitored according to the standards of Good Manufacturing Practices, often referred to as GMP. There is also the United States Pharmacopeia (USP), a pharmaceutical reference that suggests standards for the purity of water used in pharmaceutical preparations through the "Purified Water" monograph of the USP; purified water is often referred to as "aqua" in the labels of skin care products.

Water is essential to skin care formulas, in which it acts as a solvent for many ingredients and an essential component of the aqueous phase of emulsions. It is preferable that water carry as few dissolved substances as possible, because this will increase its inertia toward the formulation and lessen the risks of interaction (such as chelation) with other molecules. That is why purified and distilled water are preferred.

Water is a key ingredient for most of the formulas listed in this book. It can be added as is or used to make herbal teas or hydrosols, or simply to rinse off a mask or a scrub. Purified water and distilled water are the least likely to interfere with the products because they do not carry dissolved substances and have no harsh chlorine residue. Having a filter that can transform tap water into purified water is very convenient. It is possible to verify the level of water purity by using a total dissolved substances meter; if the reading is 0, or close to 0, that means that your water has virtually no inclusions.

Second best is spring water. Even though it is relatively high in dissolved substances, some of those dissolved substances are skin-friendly minerals such as calcium and magnesium. Another advantage is that spring water is not chlorinated.

Filtered tap water is a third choice, since most domestic filters only remove chlorine smell and heavy metals. Filtered water is better than plain tap water, but it is not as pure as purified or distilled water.

Thermal water is a unique kind of water used in particular cosmetic brands, which often own thermal water sites or stations, such as Vichy and Avène. Even though it has been extensively analyzed, this kind of water remains nonreproducible. Thermal water is linked to volcanic springs; thus the emerging water has a notably higher temperature than the average temperature of the surrounding air. Thermal water has been praised for its healing properties.

People with arthritis and other inflammatory conditions may find great benefit in bathing in thermal water springs, and that is why there are special on-site spas that offer services for various ailments, including special care for irritated, psoriatic, and atopic skin. Thermal water composition is exceptional because of all the minerals and oligo elements (trace minerals) the water collects before surfacing. Avène water, for instance, reaches the surface only after forty years of traveling below ground.

Buy or order your thermal water spray bottle online and add it to your beauty regimen to soothe, regenerate, and protect sensitive skin.

Vegetable Oils

Vegetable oils are oils from vegetable sources, obtained from specific parts of oil-bearing plants such as seeds, fruits, or roots. Vegetable oils are known as fixed oils, because, unlike essential oils, they are nonvolatile, meaning they do not evaporate. They may also be referred to as carrier oils, because they often serve as vehicles and diluting agents for essential oils. Although most vegetable oils could be applied undiluted, they are often part of a blend or are incorporated into a formula in which they make up most of the oil phase alongside butters and waxes.

Vegetable oils are extremely beneficial for skin and offer multiple benefits, such as improving skin texture, preserving moisture, preventing wrinkles, and protecting skin from environmental stressors.

Even though many vegetable oils are known for their broad cosmetic use, a lot of them are also culinary or gourmet oils; examples are olive oil, hazelnut oil, avocado oil, and sesame oil. Also, because of their packed benefits, some of them are taken internally as supplements to improve general health or aid in alleviating certain medical conditions, such as using evening primrose oil to treat menopause symptoms.

EXTRACTION METHODS

Whether they are destined for culinary use (food grade) or cosmetic formulations (cosmetic grade), it is important to inquire about the extraction method of these oils. The use of heat as part of the hydraulic extraction process can jeopardize the polyunsaturated acids in the oil and expose them to oxidation, thus stripping them of their benefits. Also, the use of solvents such as hexane or rubbing alcohol can contaminate the final product and yield less pure oil.

Cold- and expeller-pressed oils are preferred, because the oil is unaltered and its properties better preserved. Expeller-pressing methods do elevate oil temperature but not enough to threaten the oil's quality. Nevertheless, "cold-pressed" remains the gold standard and is the best method of oil extraction.

Refining is another process that can alter the state of the final oil. It employs various methods, such as flash heating, winterization, and deodorization, to produce a refined oil that has altered properties.

Most vegetable oils called for in this book are available at local grocery stores, specialty shops, and online. You can use a garlic press to extract tiny amounts of oil from nuts such as almonds, walnuts, and hazelnuts.

COMMONLY USED VEGETABLE OILS

Açaí Oil

Açaí is a berry-like fruit produced by South American acai palm trees, *Euterpe oleracea*. The oil is rich in antioxidants and key elements that play important roles in skin metabolism, such as anthocyanins, phytosterols, phenols, and vitamins B, C, and E. The main two essential fatty acids present in the oil are oleic and linoleic acids, oleic acid accounting for an average of 50 percent of the total fatty acids in the oil, and linoleic acid around 40 percent. It is also rich in essential amino acids and minerals such as iron, calcium, phosphorus, and potassium. A very generous source of antioxidants, it is indicated to prevent free-radical formation and is especially recommended for aging skin. It penetrates skin quickly and is highly moisturizing. Açaí berry oil has anti-inflammatory properties, making it a suitable additive to creams and lotions intended for patients with eczema.

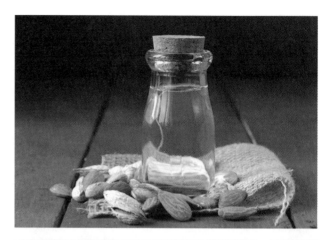

Almond Oil

Almond oil is obtained from the dry kernels of the almond, *Prunus amygdalus*. Also referred to as sweet almond oil, this light oil absorbs quickly and does not clog pores. It is suitable for most skin types and is used as a moisturizer. Found in a great number of products, almond oil is high in vitamins E and A. It is extremely rich in oleic acid (up to 86 percent) and also in linoleic acid. It is also full of antioxidants such as quercetin, quercitrin, kaempferol, and morin. Quercetin and kaempferol, in particular, are thought to offer some sun protective effects, which are an

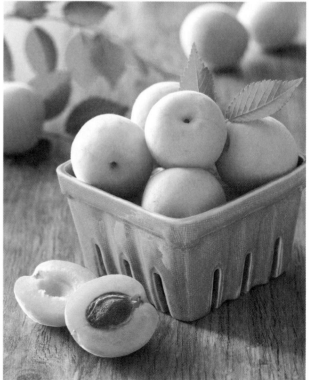

added benefit in sunscreens. Almond oil can be used as is or mixed with other oils when making skin care formulations.

Apricot Oil

Apricot oil is produced from the kernel nuts of the apricot fruit, *Prunus armeniaca*. The oil is also called apricot kernel oil. This thin oil spreads easily, absorbs quickly, and doesn't clog pores. It is rich in vitamin A, which helps fight skin aging. Oleic acid is the predominant fatty acid in apricot oil, but linoleic acid is also present in significant amounts. With uses similar to those of almond oil, it is recommended mainly for dry, mature, and sensitive skin. Use apricot oil as is or dilute with other carrier oils to a 20–50 percent ratio.

Argan Oil

Very popular in Morocco, argan oil comes from the kernels of the rare argan tree, *Argania spinosa*. Besides its culinary uses, it has long been incorporated into cosmetic preparations. It has many benefits for both skin and hair. This ancient staple item of the hammam (Turkish bath) tradition, as an ingredient in mud masks and soaps, is now gaining popularity all over the world although it is produced in limited quantities. Rich in skin-rejuvenating elements, argan oil is an excellent anti-aging oil; it is high in vitamin E and oleic and linoleic acids and contains squalene and carotenes. It can also help improve the appearance of scars. People with acne-prone skin should use this oil with care to avoid breakouts. Highly nourishing, argan oil adds luster and shine to dull hair.

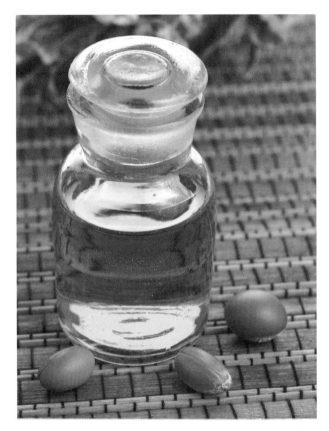

Avocado Oil

Avocado, *Persea americana*, is the richest in vitamin E, among all fruits. It is also rich in skin-benefitting fatty acids and other antioxidants. It is high in vitamins A, B1, B2, and B5. Particularly high in sterols, avocado oil is a good collagen stimulator that can also reduce the prevalence of age spots. Even though it contains much more omega-6, the omega-3 acids it contains are able to provide some protection for the skin from free radicals. It is therefore among the oils to incorporate in sunscreen formulas. It is a strong moisturizer, a powerful skin emollient that hydrates the squamous skin cells, and a powerful anti-aging oil. Because of its thick texture, avocado oil is a great choice for dehydrated and mature skin. It is also indicated for itchy skin. Even though it is well absorbed through the skin, it does leave an unpleasant greasy residue. It is therefore diluted with lighter carrier oils, such as almond oil, to a final concentration of 10–20 percent, avocado to almond oil.

Black Raspberry Seed Oil

From the seeds of the black raspberry fruit, *Rubus occidentalis*, this greenish, cold-pressed oil is a great source of antioxidants and has an interesting composition of essential fatty acids: 85 percent of the oil is essential fatty acids, 30 percent of which is the highly prized omega-3. This is a dry oil that absorbs quickly and does not clog pores. Extremely rich in various phytonutrients and antioxidants, it contains four kinds of vitamin E: alpha and gamma tocopherols, in addition to beta and gamma tocotrienols. Although

it could be used undiluted, the recommended usage level is 1–5 percent concentration, especially for mature skin to fight the signs of aging.

Blackberry Seed Oil

Pressed from the seeds of blackberry fruits, *Rubus fruticosus*, blackberry seed oil is rich in vitamin C, a skin-rejuvenating vitamin and a skin brightener. It also contains other antioxidants, such as vitamin E, phytosterols such as beta sitosterol, and both lutein and zeaxanthin. The oil is up to 90 percent unsaturated fatty acids, 20 percent of which is omega-3. Blackberry seed oil is mostly recommended for blemished, sun-damaged skin, as well as for aging skin to prevent wrinkles. It has the advantage of being stable and can be included in serums and creams with a typical concentration of 1–5 percent.

Blackcurrant Seed Oil

Blackcurrant seed oil is obtained from the seeds of *Ribes nigrum*, also known as cassis. This oil can contain up to 20 percent omega-6 polyunsaturated

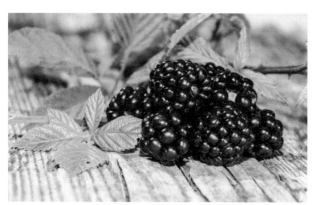

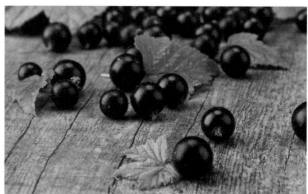

fatty acids, as well as up to 14 percent omega-3 polyunsaturated fatty acids. Blackcurrant seed oil is recommended to rejuvenate thinning hair and has anti-inflammatory properties that calm dry, scaly skin. Typical concentration is 1–5 percent.

Blueberry Seed Oil

From the seeds of *Vaccinium corymbosum*, this powerful oil is very rich in antioxidants that help protect skin from free radicals, sun damage, and aging. It can be used at a 1–5 percent concentration and is a great oil to include in facial serums.

Borage Seed Oil

Borago officinalis seeds are the highest in gamma linolenic acid (up to 24 percent of the oil), an unsaturated fatty acid that helps prevent sun damage and fights premature skin aging. This oil also contains a number of precious vitamins and minerals. Mix with other carrier oils and use at a 5–10 percent dilution for regeneration of mature skin.

Camelina Oil

From *Camelina sativa*, this oil is often referred to as "false flax" or "wild flax," but it has the advantage of being more stable than flax seed oil. Camelina oil is rich in vitamins, omega-3 polyunsaturated fatty acids (mainly ALA), and antioxidants. It is used for both skin and hair.

Camellia Seed Oil

This tea oil, from *Camellia oleifera*, is light and absorbs quickly into the skin. It is high in oleic acid (up to 85 percent) and is especially recommended for dry, mature skin. It is suitable for most skin types, including acne-prone and sensitive skin. Rich in antioxidants, it is also a beneficial oil for nails and hair. You could think of it as part of an after-sun oil or even a makeup remover. Recommended usage is in a 2–12 percent dilution.

Carrot Oil

Carrot oil is extracted from the carrot plant, *Daucus carota*. It is rich in vitamin E and carotenes, beta-car-

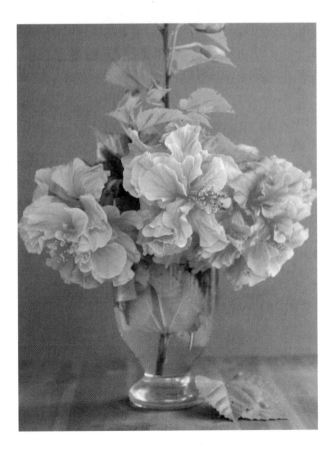

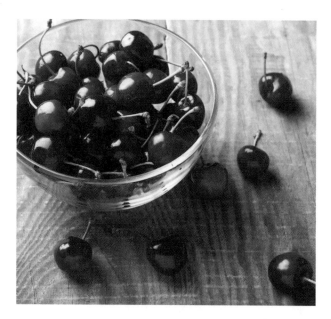

otene being a precursor of vitamin A, which is proven to help skin appear younger, minimizing the appearance of wrinkles. Dilute carrot oil with other oils to a 2–5 percent final concentration and limit its use during pregnancy.

Castor Oil

From castor beans (*Ricinus communis*), castor oil is extremely rich in the monounsaturated fatty acid ricinoleic acid. Even though the thick, somewhat sticky texture of this oil is not cosmetically appealing, castor oil has some benefits to offer: It is a powerful humectant and anti-aging oil and is also thought to promote healthier, fuller, and longer eyelashes. It is also considered by many as a good treatment for healing skin blemishes, improving the appearance of scars, and reducing skin discoloration. This oil has toxic properties; when ingested, it acts as a powerful laxative

and is contraindicated during pregnancy. Use diluted with other carrier oils to improve its cosmetic appeal.

Cherry Seed Oil

From the seeds of cherries, *Prunus cerasus*, this oil is very similar in properties to almond and apricot kernel oil. It is high in oleic acid and vitamins A and E. Cherry seed oil is a gentle moisturizer that can provide generous amounts of antioxidants. It is particularly recommended for oily skin where some astringency is useful. Research suggests that cherry seed oil can protect skin from sun damage, which is why it is an added benefit when included in sunscreen formulations.

Coconut Oil

From the coconut tree, *Cocos nucifer*, this edible oil is gaining popularity due to its many benefits for both skin and body. Pure virgin coconut oil liquifies when applied to the skin and is quickly absorbed without clogging pores. It is said to have antimicrobial properties. It is also rich in antioxidants and possesses anti-aging properties.

Cranberry Seed Oil

From the seeds of *Vaccinium macrocarpon*, this very rich oil is reported to have the highest content of vitamin E among vegetable oils. It also has a high content of omega-3 and omega-6 polyunsaturated fatty acids and is rich in phytosterols (which help lower cholesterol when ingested in foods). Phytosterols can help slow collagen destruction and even promote new collagen formation. This oil also contains vitamin A, which helps rejuvenate skin and tame wrinkles.

Cranberry seed oil is high in antioxidants; it provides protection from UV-induced free radicals and is a powerful skin moisturizer. It has medium texture and absorbs quickly. Recommended usage is in a 5 percent dilution, though some formulations could contain more. It can also be added to hair care products to strengthen and moisturize hair. Because of its more stable shelf life, it can be added to other oils to increase their stability.

Cucumber Seed Oil

From the seeds of *Cucumis sativus*, this oil is rich in phytosterols, which protect the skin's elasticity and preserve the lipid barrier, thus promoting a better-moisturized skin. Cucumber oil is high in vitamin E, which acts as an antioxidant and fights free radicals. It helps achieve more youthful skin, with a reduction in wrinkles. Linoleic acid is more predominant (up to 60 percent) in this oil than oleic acid and other polyunsaturated acids. Cucumber seed oil is recommended for aging skin, as well as for dry, irritated skin. Use it in a 10–25 percent concentration to moisturize, soothe sunburns, and prevent stretch marks.

Evening Primrose Oil

From the flower *Oenothera biennis*, this medicinal plant has benefits to offer in many areas, including premenstrual syndrome, menopausal hot flashes, chronic headaches, and migraines. Very close to borage seed oil, evening primrose oil is extremely rich in GLA (gamma linolenic acid, up to 9 percent), which is responsible for most of the benefits it offers. At the skin level, evening primrose oil provides anti-aging

effects and helps clear rosacea and acne. This oil is especially recommended for mature skin, as well as for irritated skin. It can also contribute to healthier hair and nails.

Flaxseed Oil

This oil comes from the seeds of the flax plant, *Linum usitatissimum*. Numerous properties are associated with this increasingly popular oil, whether it is used internally (ingested) or externally (on hair and skin). Flaxseed oil is high in omega-3 ALA, an essential fatty acid. The content of ALA in flaxseed oil ranges from 52 percent to 63 percent and is therefore the highest among vegetable oils. This oil has anti-inflammatory properties and is an important ingredient for aging skin. Flax seeds contain lignans, a type of phytoestrogen known to have antioxidant properties. Extraction of the oil can contribute to the loss of those lignans unless they are added at the end of the process. Flaxseed oil is highly susceptible to oxidation; thus, adding it to formulations requires preservation with other antioxidants such as vitamin E. It becomes rancid within weeks, store it in the refrigerator to slow its oxidation.

Grape Seed Oil

From the seeds of *Vitis vinifera*, the common grape vine, this thin oil is rich in antioxidants. It absorbs quickly and is therefore a good choice for oily skin and whenever oily residues are to be avoided. It can be used full strength or diluted with other oils. Add it to facial serums and other skin preparations at a 1–3 percent level. It makes a good base for preparations when nut allergies are a concern.

Hazelnut Oil

Pressed from the seeds of *Corylus avellana*, this astringent oil is one of the best oils for acne-prone skin. It is also thought to be beneficial for thread veins. Recommended mainly for oily skin types, it can be incorporated into formulas with a 10 percent dilution, up to 100 percent of the oily phase. It is also added to many sunscreens because it may have sun-filtering capability.

Hemp Seed Oil

This oil comes from the plant *Cannabis sativa*. With a composition similar to that of the skin's natural lipids, this dry oil is light and leaves no thick, oily film when applied. Because it is very rich in polyunsaturated acids (80 percent), it needs to be stored in dark or amber bottles away from sunlight and heat to protect those unsaturated acids from oxidation and thus spoilage of the oil. Hemp seed oil is especially recommended for dry and mature skin. It can be used for as low as 2.5 percent of your formulation; increasing the concentration to 10 percent will generate more benefits for the skin.

Jojoba Oil

Pressed from the seeds of the jojoba plant, *Simmondsia chinensis*, this golden oil resembles natural skin oils. It is low in polyunsaturated fatty acids and high in tocopherols (vitamin E), which helps it resist rancidity and why it is preferred among carrier oils. Its properties are those of both an oil and a liquid wax, and it is sometimes referred to as liquid wax.

This skin-friendly oil is a good choice for all skin types. It improves skin softness and moisture and can

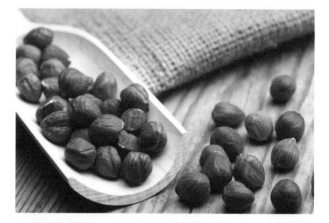

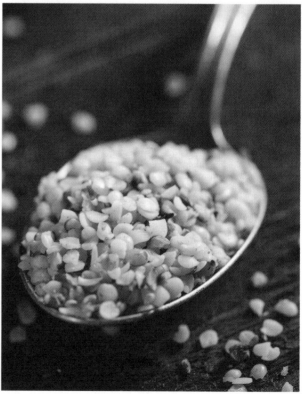

help reduce fine lines. It is a great addition to both skin and hair products. It can be used as a 100 percent oil base or diluted to lesser concentrations. It is specifically recommended for acne-prone skin, because it helps balance skin oils and break down sebum in clogged pores. It also makes a good base for scalp oils.

Kukui Nut Tree Oil

This oil is not very popular around the world but has long provided the inhabitants of Hawaii Island with numerous benefits. The kukui nuts from *Aleurites moluccana*, known as the candlenut tree, among other names, are pressed to obtain this oil. Rich in linoleic acid and ALA, the oil is a great moisturizer, helping relieve chapped skin and minimize skin irritation.

Macadamia Oil

This oil is pressed from the nuts of the macadamia tree, *Macadamia integrifolia*. It is stable because of its high content of monounsaturated fatty acids. It is high in palmitoleic acid, which gives it antioxidative properties. It absorbs quickly, protects skin, and is beneficial for scar reduction and sunburns. This regenerative oil is suitable for dry, mature skin, as well as for all skin types.

Neem Oil

This oil comes from the neem plant, *Azadirachta indica*. It is used in hair preparations to strengthen hair and improve shine. This strongly scented oil is also used for its antibacterial, antiparasitic, and insect repellent powers.

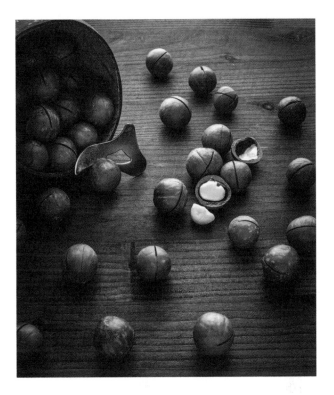

Olive Oil

Cold pressed from the fruits of the olive tree, *Olea europaea*, this Mediterranean edible oil is also a great asset in making beauty products. Because it is a little thicker than other oils, it is more suitable for dry skin. It is high in oleic acid, absorbs quickly yet allows the skin to breathe, and doesn't clog pores. Rich in the antioxidant, anti-aging vitamin E and vitamin A, olive oil is beneficial as a skin softener, moisturizer, and soother for irritated skin. Use it undiluted as massage oil or incorporate it into your formulations at a 10 percent ratio.

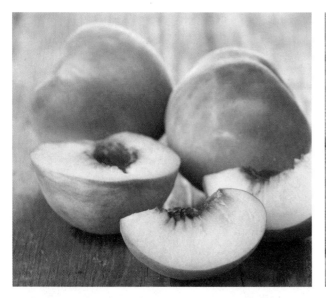
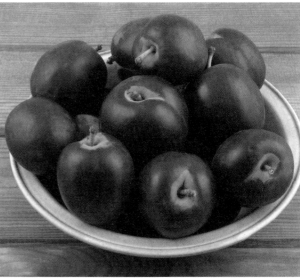

Peach Kernel Oil

Extracted from the kernels of peaches, *Prunus persica*, peach kernel oil is very close to apricot kernel oil. It also makes a valid substitute for almond oil or grape seed oil. Use undiluted or include in your formulations at a 5–10 percent ratio.

Plum Kernel Oil

This oil comes from the kernels of plums, *Prunus domestica*. This golden oil is rich in vitamins E and A and antioxidants. Oleic and linoleic acids are the two most prevalent fatty acids of this oil. Its uses are similar to those of almond and apricot kernel oils.

Pomegranate Seed Oil

This oil is obtained from the seeds of the pomegranate fruit, *Punica granatum*. It is a dry oil that absorbs quickly. Pomegranate is a well-known source of antioxidants, and so is its oil. It makes a great addition to sunscreen formulations and whenever anti-aging

properties are needed. Use at a 10 percent ratio in your formulations, especially when they are destined for dry, mature skin, as well as for irritated, sun-damaged skin.

Pumpkin Seed Oil

From the seeds of pumpkin, *Curcubita pepo*, this "green gold" oil is rich in vitamins A and C and in zinc. It is also a great source of omega-3 and omega-6 polyunsaturated fatty acids, mainly linoleic and oleic acid, as well as antioxidants and sterols.

Red Raspberry Seed Oil

Like most berries, raspberries, *Rubus idaeus*, are high in antioxidants. The oil has UV-filtering capabilities and is therefore a suitable oil to include in sunscreens. It is also rich in the antioxidant vitamin E, as well as the rejuvenating vitamin A. Red raspberry oil is also a good source of polyunsaturated fatty acids such as linoleic, alpha linolenic, and oleic

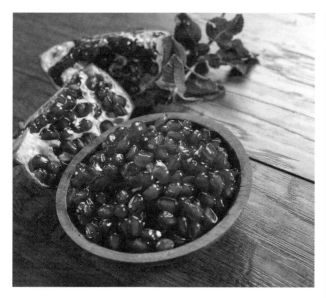

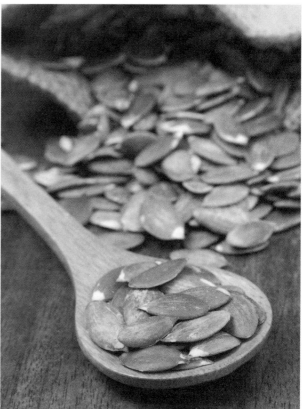

acids. Although it could be used undiluted, it is most commonly included at a 5–10 percent ratio in skin preparations.

Rice Bran Oil

This oil is obtained from the bran of the rice kernel, *Oryza sativa*. This emollient oil is used as a skin moisturizer. It is rich in vitamin E and other antioxidants. It is also capable of absorbing UV light and makes a great oil to incorporate in sunscreens. It is rich in polyunsaturated fatty acids such as oleic, linoleic, and palmitic acids. It could be used to replace nut oils when allergies are a concern. Recommended usage ratio ranges from 5 percent to 100 percent.

Rosehip Oil

This oil is obtained mainly from the seeds of wild rose bushes, *Rosa mosqueta* (also known as *Rosa rubiginosa*). This amber-colored oil is recognized as one of the richest cosmetic oils. It contains up to

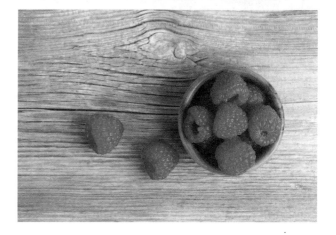

80 percent polyunsaturated fatty acids, such as linoleic and gamma linolenic acids, as well as vitamins A and C. It is also high in lycopene, which is a natural antioxidant found in tomatoes and watermelon. Rosehip oil helps with skin regeneration; improves the appearance of scars; reduces wrinkles, especially around the eyes and mouth; and protects from sun damage. It makes a good choice for dry, mature skin. It is most commonly used at a 10 percent ratio but could be used up to 100 percent, because it is very gentle and affordable.

Safflower Oil

Pressed from the seeds of the safflower plant, *Carthamus tinctorius*, this oil is extremely high in oleic and linoleic acids and makes a potent skin moisturizer. Its emollient properties prevent moisture loss from the skin surface. It is also rich in vitamin E, an antioxidant that protects skin from sun damage and prevents premature aging.

Sesame Oil

This oil is pressed from the seeds of the sesame plant, *Sesamum indicum*. Sesame oil is rich in numerous vitamins and minerals and high in vitamin E, which contributes to its anti-aging properties. It also contains the antioxidant sesamol. Sesame paste (also known as tahini) has a very high oil content and is widely used in Mediterranean cuisine, such as hummus. The oil is approved for commercial use in sunscreens because it helps block some UV rays. It is rich in polyunsaturated fatty acids, mostly linoleic acid. Use this oil in a 10–15 percent dilution, up to 100 percent. Because of the heaviness of this oil, it is usually diluted with other oils, but it can be used as is for around the eyes to reduce wrinkles and restore normal hydration.

Sunflower Oil

Cold pressed from the seeds of the sunflower, *Helianthus annus*, this oil is widely used for culinary purposes but can be very useful as a cosmetic ingredient in formulations destined for dry, weathered skin. Because it is so gentle, sunflower oil is recommended for sensitive and delicate skin. It is high in oleic acid and provides good amounts of vitamin A and E, which makes it a great oil for mature skin.

Tomato Seed Oil

From the seeds of the tomato, *Solanum lycopersicum*, this oil is very high in antioxidants, vitamins, and minerals. It also contains the antioxidant lycopene. It is especially recommended for mature, sun-damaged, and dehydrated skin types.

Walnut Oil

Pressed from walnuts, *Juglans regia*, this oil has demonstrated multiple valuable properties. It is high in polyunsaturated fatty acids, with an interesting 1:5 ratio of omega-3 to omega-6; various vitamins and minerals, such as vitamin B complex, manganese, and phosphorus; as well as a number of antioxidants. Walnut oil is an oil of choice for mature skin: It fights wrinkles, moisturizes and soothes inflammation. Recommended usage level is 10–15 percent.

Wheat Germ Oil

This oil is extracted from the germ of the common wheat plant, *Triticum vulgare*. It is exceptionally high in vitamin E, with an average content of

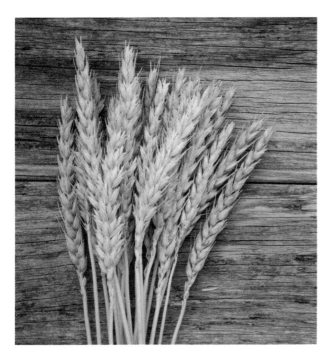

255 milligrams per 100 grams. High in linoleic acid and mixed tocopherols, this oil makes a valuable anti-aging oil. Use for cracked skin, scars, and stretch marks, between 5 and 10 percent. Avoid in cases of wheat or gluten allergies.

Flower or Herb Oils

Some vegetable oils on the market are not actually extracted from the herb or flower named but are the result of the maceration of that herb or flower in a vegetable oil that serves as a vehicle. Arnica oil, for example, is made by macerating arnica flowers in jojoba oil. Maceration will promote substance and scent transfer from the plant or flower to the oil, and the filtered final oil will offer some of the plant's original properties.

Vegetable Butters

Vegetable butters are thicker than oils and are usually solid at room temperature. Heating the butters beyond their melting point will liquefy them, allowing mixing with other ingredients. A number of butters, especially nut butters, are excellent skin moisturizers and elasticity restorers. Among the most famous are cocoa butter (used abundantly in stretch mark creams) and shea butter (used in a wide array of skin and hair products).

NATURAL BUTTERS VS. HYDROGENATED OILS

Not all butters are actually butters. A number of so-called butters are transformed oils that become solid at room temperature. Although gelation processes might be used, hydrogenation is the most commonly used commercial process for this. Hydrogen atoms saturate a number of unsaturated bonds within the molecules of the oil, which is then transformed into a more solid compound. The hydrogenation process is also used in the food industry. The resulting trans fats obtained have been linked to unfavorable health effects and are often avoided. Hydrogenated vegetable oils are, therefore, different from naturally occurring butters. Examples of hydrogenated vegetable oils include hemp seed butter, avocado butter, and sweet almond butter. The advantage of those butters over their oil form is essentially the consistency and the nice slip they can give to a facial cream or lotion. They are, however, processed and thus less "natural," by definition, than their cold-pressed oil counterparts. Hydrogenated oils may also have been refined, deodorized, and bleached.

COMMONLY USED NATURAL BUTTERS

Cocoa Butter

From the seeds of cocoa, *Theobroma cacao*, also known as the cocoa bean, comes this butter, which is rich in fatty acids and polyphenols. Unless deodorized through a special process, this solid butter has a typical chocolaty smell. Cocoa butter is well known for reducing stretch marks and improving skin elasticity and is therefore included in many pregnancy belly creams. Even though it is moisturizing, the fact that it could be comedogenic (tending to clog pores) makes it poorly recommended for facial use, especially in cases of acne-prone skin.

Kokum Butter

Kokum butter is obtained from the Indian garcinia tree, *Garcinia indica*. It has regenerative properties that help with skin healing. This astringent butter is rich in fatty acids and absorbs easily when it liquefies upon contact with the skin. Add it to your balms, soap bars, lip products, and foot care creams.

Mango Butter

From the kernels of the mango fruit, *Mangifera indica*, this rather hard butter is great for lipsticks and balms. It prevents wrinkles and dryness. Rich in fatty acids and a number of vitamins and minerals, mango butter is also beneficial for a wide array of skin conditions to nurture, soothe, and moisturize.

Murumuru Butter

This butter is obtained from the fruits of the Brazilian murumuru palm tree, *Astrocaryum murumuru*. Unlike cocoa butter, murumuru butter has a very mild smell. It is rich in essential fatty acids and vitamin A precursors. Incorporate it into your anti-aging creams and lip and body balms.

Shea Butter

Pressed from the nuts of the shea tree (*Vitellaria paradoxa*, previously called *Butyrospermum parkii*), this highly moisturizing butter is also known as karité (*beurre de karité*, in French), which means tree of life. This age-old African butter has a lot to offer: It is an excellent moisturizer, is rich in vitamins A and E, nourishes skin, and improves elasticity. It also contains a number of antioxidant phenolic compounds. Add it to your creams, balms, lotions, even hair products, for softening. Because it is noncomedogenic, it is more suitable for acne-prone skin than cocoa butter and can help improve the appearance of acne scars.

Botanicals

Numerous herbs and flowers carry multiple skin benefits. Whether used as hydrosols, powders, extracts, teas, or essential oils, they remain a strong pillar in cosmetics. Some of the recipes included in this book call for specific flower waters, also known as hydrosols, herbal teas, or herbal extracts, most of which are available at local grocery stores, specialty shops, or online. But for the enthusiasts who would like to start their product from as close to scratch as possible, and possibly grow their own organic herbs and flowers, the methodology of making your own hydrosols and herbal extracts follows, beginning with a few points about harvesting:

- Make sure you identify and collect the right part of the plant—for example, petals versus buds.

- Pick your flowers and herbs on sunny days after morning dew has evaporated, to keep humidity at its lowest and help preserve your plants.

- If you are after essential oils, pick your flowers early in the morning when the concentration is at its peak and before the warm sun triggers evaporation.

- Avoid "older" plants because of potential insect and parasite exposure.

- While flower buds are best picked in the spring, leaves are at their best prior to blooming.

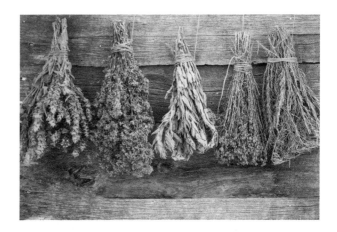

DRYING HERBS AND FLOWERS

You can dry delicate, fragile, and small leaves and plants as they are. Chop larger herbs into smaller pieces for easier and faster drying. Do not wash herbs or flowers prior to drying them, because excess humidity will encourage mold and other parasitic growth.

The simplest way to dry your herbs is to spread them on a paper towel and place it in a ventilated cool area away from direct sunlight, heat, and humidity. As days go by, the herbs will start to lose their moisture and wilt. Avoiding excess heat and direct sunlight is of crucial importance, especially if the herbs contain essential oils that could be lost in such conditions. You can tell that your herbs are dry enough when you can easily turn them into powder by rubbing a small quantity between the palms of your hands. If you need powdered herbs, use a mortar and pestle to pulverize your plant. A coffee grinder is a time saver for bigger quantities.

Another way to dry your herbs is to spread a thin layer on a porous foil sheet and place it on a wire rack in the oven. Simply puncture the surface of the foil with a fork or toothpick to let air circulate and allow more uniform drying of the herbs. Keep oven temperature at the lowest setting possible. Overheating your plants might alter the nature of the botanicals you are after. This method is more suitable for heat-tolerant parts of plants such as roots.

When your herbs are dry, store them, up to two years, in amber glass jars away from heat, humidity, and sunlight. Do not forget the labels: Write down the name of the plant and the date it was harvested.

HOW TO MAKE YOUR OWN INFUSIONS, DECOCTIONS, AND HYDROSOLS

Making an infusion, or herbal infusion, is comparable to making tea: Just pour boiling water over the loose herbs or herbal tea bag and cover with a lid. Steeping time might vary, but 15 minutes is usually enough. Wait until the infusion has reached room temperature before filtering or removing the herbal tea bag to ensure maximum benefit. Using powdered plants is not recommended for infusions, because filtering might become difficult, resulting in a cloudy suspension.

Decoction is different and is a more powerful extraction, since water and plant boil simultaneously. While it can be aggressive toward essential oils and flower petals, it is the best extraction method for roots. The average recommended boiling time is 30 minutes, and, of course, cooling time is essential prior to an application.

In general, infusion is the method of choice for flowers, leaves, and other "fragrant" parts of the plant; decoction is more suitable for thicker parts, such as tree bark and roots.

Hydrosols are sometimes referred to as flower waters and are usually a commercially obtained by-product of steam distillation yielding essential oils. An example is rose water.

Flower waters can be obtained through the infusion technique explained above. The usual ratio is 1 part flower to 10 parts water, unless otherwise indicated. It is important not to boil flowers or petals because of the fragile nature of their components; stirring occasionally can be beneficial to promote substance transfer. When the hydrosol reaches room temperature, it can be filtered and transferred to a bottle with a lid. If it will be stored for later use, labeling it with the name of the flower and the preparation date will prevent confusion and using it after it has expired.

MAKING YOUR OWN HERBAL EXTRACTS AND TINCTURES

Herbal extracts are important ingredients that enrich many skin product formulations and offer valuable benefits such as anti-aging and skin-brightening effects. They are much more concentrated than hydrosols and bring much less water content to the formula; extracts have the advantage of offering their benefits via a dropper.

Obtaining herbal extracts has become part of modern industrial science. Different solvents and various techniques are employed to extract concentrated "goodness" from plants. New extracts are introduced regularly, and even if they might be a little expensive, they do take beauty products to a different level. Some examples follow:

- Anti-aging extracts, including edelweiss, watermelon, blueberry, alfalfa, and algae.

- Skin-brightening extracts, such as licorice, lemon, grapefruit, and other vitamin C–containing extracts.

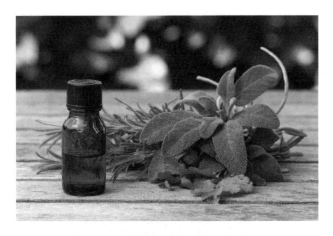

- Extracts with sun protection properties, such as rice bran and cranberry seed.

Many herbal extracts need to be refrigerated, and all of them need to be diluted; generally, 1–5 percent is the recommended level, depending on the nature of the extract. Follow your supplier's recommendations.

Even though most extracts are commercially available, it is possible to extract small quantities at home with very little equipment. The process is often less expensive than buying commercially and allows you to choose your own preferred solvent.

Rubbing alcohol is widely used as a solvent, because it is a powerful extracting agent and stores well; tinctures are extractions made with rubbing alcohol as a solvent. Because herbal extracts are diluted with the remaining ingredients of an earlier preparation, the residual amount of alcohol is insignificant.

It is best to start with fresh and organic herbs. Fresh herbs have not had time to lose precious substances and are, therefore, capable of yielding a better-quality extract; organically grown herbs are preferred if you want to avoid pesticides. Wait for your herbs to start to wilt before proceeding with extraction; lay the harvested plant on paper towels and leave it in a cool area, away from direct sunlight. The purpose is not to dry the plant but just to get rid of excess moisture, which is achievable within a day or two, depending on the plant. If fresh herbs are not available, dried herbs might be used instead; just avoid powdered ones, because filtration will be harder and the resulting extract might be cloudy.

Start by chopping the herbs and putting them in a glass container with a tight lid. Pour high-proof alcohol or vodka over the herbs. Use 3 parts alcohol to 1 part herbs. If you are using dried herbs, add more alcohol (up to 5 parts total), because dried herbs will absorb some of the alcohol. Put on the lid and put the jar away from sunlight and heat. Shake two to three times daily. After three to five days, use a coffee filter or a cheesecloth to filter and strain the solution. Squeeze the herbs to get the last drop (this is the most concentrated part, which you definitely want). Filter again if needed.

Further concentration of the extract can be achieved by repeating the same process with another batch of herbs using the same alcohol. Usually, the darker the extract color, the more concentrated it is. Pour the extract into an amber bottle and store in a cool place. Make sure you label the bottle with

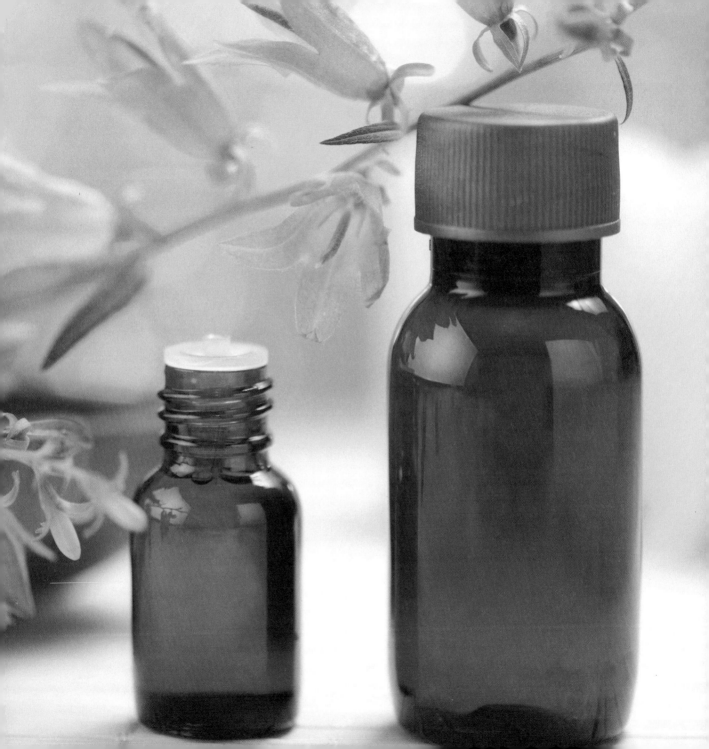

the herbal extract name and the date you made it. Because this is an alcoholic preparation, tinctures should remain good to use for up to three years. Make sure to shake the extract prior to using it to disperse suspended particles.

Essential Oils

Essential oils are highly fragrant, super concentrated, and extremely volatile; and their effects on humans are proven and documented. Even though a growing number of synthetic fragrances are available at much cheaper prices, manufacturers still rely on essential oils when making more natural products that are less sensitizing and have better skin tolerability.

EXTRACTION

Steam distillation is often the method of choice for extracting essential oils. It takes a lot of flowers to yield a little essential oil. Even though some highly fragrant flowers contain more essential oil, very large amounts are needed for extraction—for example, two pounds of petals produce only one ounce of essential oil.

ESSENTIAL OILS METHODOLOGY

Essential oils and extracts are extremely concentrated and should be diluted before they are applied to the skin. In general, for cosmetic purposes, essential oils should not exceed twelve drops per ounce of finished product. If unsure, stay within the 1 percent limit. Use a quarter of that amount if pregnant, and even less or none at all if the product is intended for babies.

Because the scent of an essential oil can be potentially disturbing and maybe hazardous in some cases, it is important to be in a well-ventilated area when using them. They are also volatile and flammable and should not be inhaled or applied undiluted.

A health hazard might be posed by some essential oils, including arnica, onion, garlic, camphor, mustard, sassafras, rue, pennyroyal, horseradish, wormwood, sweet birch, bitter almond, wintergreen, and others. Eugenol, for example, which is present in clove, can be toxic to the liver at high concentrations. It is, therefore, important to read package inserts and research safety precautions pertaining to specific essential oils before working with them in cosmetics or in aromatherapy.

CHOOSING ESSENTIAL OILS

Choose your essential oils according to your taste or mood. Essential oils can improve the smell of your product and uplift your spirit at the same time. A little reading on aromatherapy will help you know which essential oils will interest you. Tangerine, grapefruit, and lemon are widely used citrusy essential oils, especially in personal care products. They can be photosensitizing when added to facial creams, so the use of sunscreen with them is recommended. Flower-derived essential oils, such as gardenia and geranium, are also very popular—or even rose and jasmine, which remain among the most expensive essential oils. Other deeper scents, such as cedar and sandalwood, are more popular in the perfume industry.

Essential oils that may have an astringent effect—mainly tea tree, neem, and neroli—are preferred for acne-prone skin. Some studies have shown that tea tree oil can improve acne through two different mechanisms: its antiseptic effect, which counteracts bacterial proliferation on the skin surface, and its astringent effect, which helps reduce sebum production. It is also more skin friendly and causes less irritation and dryness than acne medications.

Neem essential oil has antiseptic properties that help to clear skin. It prevents infection of clogged pores and assists in the healing of infected cysts.

Both neroli essential oil and neroli water are astringent and can reduce sebum production.

ABSOLUTES AND CO2S

Absolutes and CO2 extracts are also highly fragrant extracts that have some differences with essential oils. Absolutes are even more concentrated than essential oils but might contain residual amounts of the solvents used during the extraction process. CO2s are thought to be better than essential oils because pressurized CO2 will evaporate after extraction, leaving a thicker essential oil with a less altered fragrance. Steam-distilled essential oils are still the most popular and have great potency and high purity.

FLOWER OILS

Because essential oils can be costly and difficult to obtain, flower oils might be a more convenient and affordable alternative. Flower oils are made by adding highly fragrant flowers to a neutral oil such as sun-flower oil and allowing enough time for substances such as essential oils to be transferred from the flowers to the vehicle oil. Part of the essential oils within the flowers will be diluted within the oil used, and that is why flower oils can smell like essential oils, while being a much less expensive alternative. Flower oils are not as concentrated as essential oils, and that is why a much larger quantity is usually called for.

PRESERVATIVES

Preservatives have become a sensitive topic because of the controversy associated with the use of synthetic preservatives. First of all, it needs to be clearly stated that all commercial skin care products, natural or not, must be preserved in an adequate and efficient manner. Creams, lotions, and gels contain large amounts of water, which makes them susceptible to the growth of microorganisms and to spoilage. They require adequate preservation that guarantees their usage safety up to a certain period of time.

Synthetic preservatives, such as parabens, phenoxyethanol, sodium benzoate, and potassium sorbate, are efficient at low concentrations and are used in a wide array of personal care products, pharmaceutical products, and various foods. However, because of the increasing doubt in their safety profile, some of them (mainly parabens) are being phased out of many commercial products. Food companies have taken similar steps and removed or substituted some of the synthetic preservatives that were part of the ingredients.

The challenge that the "natural products" industry is currently facing is being able to replace

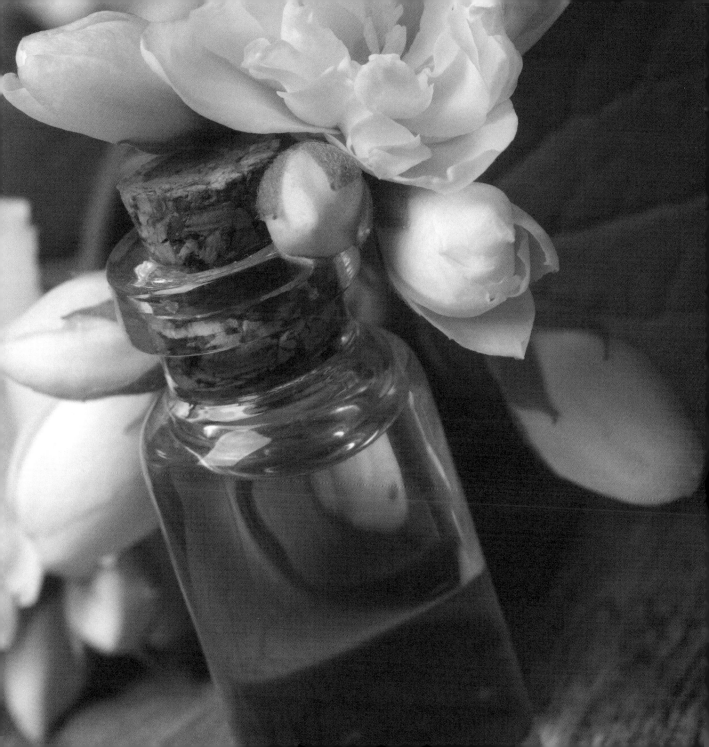

those highly efficient preservatives with new equally effective and less questionable preserving agents. While homemade beauty products are designed for personal and immediate use and rarely need preservatives, commercial cosmetics need to rely on a concoction of natural extracts and botanicals.

Those preservatives should be able to ensure a sufficient shelf life for the products and protect them from deterioration and spoilage. Natural preservatives do exist and are efficient, especially if used in the right concentrations. Manufacturers often use more than one preservative to achieve this objective. Auxiliary techniques, such as using amber or dark blue glass containers and UV-filtering bottles to minimize photo oxidation and extend shelf life, are also implemented.

Natural Preservatives

Going natural does not mean avoiding ingredients; it just means using natural ones. There are many effective all-natural preservatives available online or maybe at your local vitamin store.

The most natural preservatives that you can add to your beauty products are grape seed extract (GSE), tea tree essential oil, rosemary oil or rosemary oil extract, vitamin E, and pomegranate seed oil. Check the product specificities for adequate concentration range. For most of them, a 0.5 percent level will provide a reasonable extension of the shelf life of your finished product. Rosemary oil extract is effective at 0.1 percent concentration. You can use one at a time, or maybe even build your own blend of preservatives.

NATURE IDENTICAL PRESERVATIVES

Producers need to ensure the microbiological safety of their products. Preserving products with purely natural ingredients is often difficult and requires elaborate expertise. "Nature-identical" preservatives are often permitted, but their use must be clearly indicated on the product packaging, guaranteeing transparency for the consumer.

T-50 Vitamin E Oil

Vitamin E, or tocopherol, is a natural antioxidant that can extend the life of skin care products. Gamma tocopherol, a component of vitamin E, is a great antioxidant for protecting cosmetic formulations. Use at 0.04 percent to protect your formulations or check supplier's instructions, as tocopherol concentrations vary.

Rosemary Oil Extract

From *Rosmarinus officinalis* leaves, this extract, known as ROE, also acts as a natural antioxidant. ROE can impart its own aroma and affect the final odor of the product. As a preservative, add 0.15–0.5 percent if undiluted.

Grapefruit Seed Extract

Grapefruit seed extract (GSE) is a popular antimicrobial widely used as a natural preservative in skin care products. It is obtained from grapefruit seeds and pulp. It is often sold diluted with vegetable glycerin to minimize skin irritation when added to various skin formulations. The usual commercial ratio is ⅓ GSE in ⅔ glycerin, but this can vary between sup-

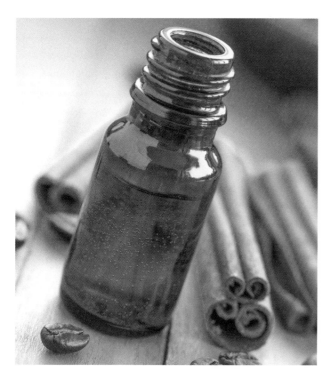

monly used as preservatives in food, pharmaceutical, and cosmetic preparations.

Sorbic acid (E200), sodium sorbate (E201), potassium sorbate (E202), and calcium sorbate (E203) are antimicrobials that can inhibit the growth of fungi, yeast, and mold. They are considered to be safe for humans and do not accumulate in the environment. The usual concentration for cosmetics preservation ranges between 0.15 and 0.3 percent.

HOMEMADE SKINCARE PRODUCTS PRESERVATION

When you are making your own skin care products, you will most likely use them up before they have time to spoil. Prepare small batches and store them adequately, in small-opening jars or dispensing bottles, away from sunlight, heat, and humidity, which would promote unwanted chemical reactions within your product, as well as bacterial and fungal growth. You can further protect your formulations by adding one or more of the natural preservatives mentioned above.

Dry (anhydrous) formulations, such as balms and oils, do not require preservatives if sealed and stored as recommended. Salves and balms are usually rich in vitamin E, which acts as an antioxidant, preventing rancidity and protecting the oils.

Bath bombs, scrub salts, soap bars, and bath and massage oils do not need preservatives. Just add a little extra vitamin E to protect the oils from oxidation and store the preparation in a dry place away from humidity. Store your oils in amber bottles, tightly sealed, and away from heat and humidity.

pliers. The recommended usage level ranges between 0.5 and 1.0 percent.

Essential Oils

Even though a number of essential oils are known to have some antimicrobial activity, the concentration required is more than what can be added to cosmetics. Examples are caraway, cinnamon, clove, cumin, eucalyptus, lavender, lemon, rose, rosemary, sage, sandalwood, and thyme.

Sorbates

Sorbates are the salts of the naturally occurring sorbic acid. They are synthetically produced and com-

Emollients and Humectants

Glycerin remains the most widely used ingredient in these products and has multiple applications, including food, pharmaceutical, and industrial usages. This polyol is an alcohol in nature. It is water soluble and hygroscopic, which means that it attracts water. This property, together with its low toxicity, has contributed to its vast use in cosmetics. It is an emollient, a skin soother, and a powerful solvent. It is thicker than water and has a consistency similar to that of simple syrup. Because it is colorless and odorless, incorporating it into cosmetics does not affect the color or the smell of the finished product. It is also widely used as a solvent in perfumery. Glycerin is a by-product of soap making and can therefore be of animal or vegetable source. Petroleum-sourced glycerin is usually darker than nonpetroleum-derived glycerin. Vegetable glycerin is usually the preferred choice for natural skin care.

Thickeners

A number of thickeners are included in creams and lotions to provide them with adequate texture and improve stability.

CLAYS

Clays are naturally rich in minerals, exfoliate skin, and take away toxins and excess oils. That is why most clays are great for oily skin. They also give body and texture to beauty mixes and are part of all spa regimens around the world. Kaolin, bentonite, illite, Moroccan rassoul, and French green are all good examples of cosmetic clays. Unlike technical clays, cosmetic-grade clays should be very low in lead content. If you have dry skin, choose a clay that is appropriate for your skin type, such as yellow kaolin, which does not wash away skin oils.

GUMS

Gums are usually powders obtained from various sources and have a wide range of applications mainly in the food and cosmetics industries, where they act as rheology modifiers, thickeners, and stabilizers.

Guar gum is a natural powder obtained from guar, or cluster, beans (*Cyamopsis tetragonolobus*).

Gum arabic crystals are obtained from acacia trees, and this kind of gum is sometimes called acacia gum.

Xanthan gum is secreted by bacteria called Xanthomonas campestris and is widely used in food and cosmetics. It is added to warm liquids, around 100–105°F to thicken them. It is recommended to start with 0.3 percent weight ratio of xanthan gum and then increase by 0.1 percent increments until you reach the right consistency. Usually, ¼–½ teaspoon per cup of liquid will provide noticeable thickening. Using too much can lead to a slimy and stringy texture. Xanthan gum can be hydrated (mixed with a small amount of liquid) 15 minutes prior to incorporation into the liquid for an easier mixing.

CELLULOSE

Mainly obtained from wood pulp and cotton, cellulose and cellulose derivatives have a broad array of uses, ranging from food additives to cosmetic ingredients as rheology modifiers and stability enhancers.

STARCH

Abundant in many foods, including corn, rice, potatoes, and wheat, starch is less crystalline than cellulose. It is also widely used in cosmetics as a binder and thickener.

Emulsifiers

Emulsions are a dispersion of an oily phase within an aqueous phase, or an aqueous phase within an oily phase. Creams and lotions are emulsions. Emulsifiers prevent separation or settling and make the emulsion more stable. However, even if you do achieve a stable emulsion, it might be too runny. Adding a thickener will help you achieve a more luxurious texture that is both pleasant and stable. Many ingredients can be both emulsifying and thickening agents.

Beeswax is a natural emulsifier and a good thickener (upon solidification). Usually, 1 part beeswax to 4 parts oil will yield a rather firm balm. Adding more oil can give a softer balm. Carnauba wax is also a natural thickener and can work as a vegan alternative to beeswax. It is obtained from the leaves of the palm tree *Copernicia prunifera*.

Lecithin is another well-known emulsifier and occurs naturally in multiple foods such as egg yolks, soybeans, milk, fish, and others. Commercially available, lecithin is mostly obtained from soybean oil and can be sold as a powder or a liquid. It is added to creams and lotions as an emulsifier and a stabilizer.

Glyceryl stearate and stearic acid are natural emulsifying thickeners (make sure they are vegetable derived). Glyceryl stearate is the monoester of glycerin and stearic acid and is a popular oil-in-water emulsifier and thickener; its recommended usage is 2–10 percent. Stearic acid is an anionic emulsifier that has a cooling effect on skin and is usually melted and incorporated into lotions and creams also at 2–10 percent concentration. Cetyl alcohol is a thickener that can act as a co-emulsifier when used at a 5 percent or greater concentration.

pH Adjusters

Citric acid and baking soda are often used to adjust the final pH of a product and meet the skin's normal pH. Even though skin pH can vary greatly, with reports ranging from 4 to 7, it is believed that the average pH is slightly lower than 5 (4.7) and acidic. Baking soda is added to increase pH and make a preparation less acidic. Citric acid is often used to lower pH and make a preparation more acidic.

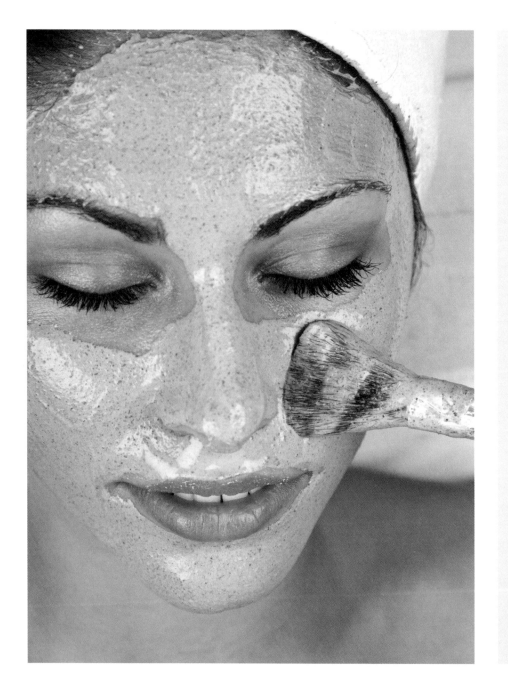

Recipes

2

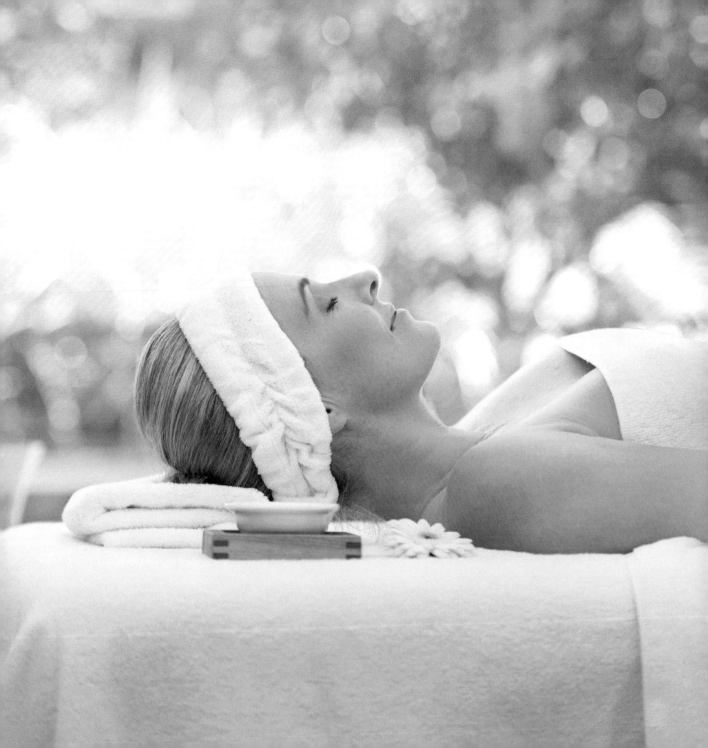

CHAPTER 4

Making Your Own Skin Care Products

With a growing demand for more natural products that are kind to both skin and body, that are effective and affordable, and whose use is clear and comprehensible, many people have found their needs met, at least partially, by homemade products.

Whether it is "just for the fun of it," to save money, or to have full control and knowledge of what goes in and what stays out, making your own skin care products remains a skillful art that translates an uncompromised passion for beauty. No matter the motive, the methodology is the same. This hobby-like science will answer multiple beauty needs with customized formulas that are effective, safe, and enjoyable.

While beginners might want to follow formulas exactly as they are presented, growing talent and practice can fuel creativity. It is important, however, to respect proportions and the whole structure of the formula.

A few basic things are essential before starting to make your own skin care products, and they are explained in the following sections of this chapter.

Work Surface

Start with a clean and well lit work surface. Your kitchen island or a part of your countertop should do. Clear a little space for your ingredients in one of your kitchen cabinets or in your basement, where it is cooler.

Ventilation is important, especially when using essential oils, as long as the circulating air is clean. Working under a hood, when available, is a valid choice, because a hood has a unidirectional airflow, meaning that it sucks away the vapors without bringing in unwelcome particles.

Basic Equipment

The utensils you need will vary somewhat with each formula. Most formulas require basic equipment, but some may call for a longer list of tools, many of which you probably already have: medium-size glass bowls, porcelain mugs, a stainless steel whisk, cheesecloth, a stick blender, a digital or kitchen scale, several pans and a stove, a spatula, small jars with lids, spray or pump bottles (recycled), rubbing alcohol (for sanitizing and disinfecting tools), lint-free towel or gauze, dropper, measuring cups and spoons, and a kitchen thermometer. A cheese grater might serve as a beeswax shaver, especially if you opt for beeswax bars rather than small pellets. It is always recommended to separate the tools you use for cooking from the ones you will be working with, to avoid cross contamination and odor transfer. Because of its lack of inertia, plastic is not the best material for making cosmetics; glass and stainless steel are better choices whenever available, especially when ingredients will be heated.

Be sure to check the formula before starting in order to have your needed utensils cleaned and ready to use.

Sanitizing

It is very important to work with sanitized utensils on a sanitized work surface and maintain proper hygiene from start to finish. This will protect the product from microbial contamination and help extend its shelf life, even with few or no preservatives.

Cleaning your work surface is crucial, as is cleaning your utensils, jars, and containers. Contamination might compromise your finished product and increase chances of quick spoilage. Begin cleaning with soap and water; then finish with rubbing alcohol and a lint-free towel. Allow time for the alcohol to evaporate completely before starting. Glass and stainless-steel utensils and containers can be sanitized in the dishwasher; wipe them with rubbing alcohol afterward for complete disinfection.

Basic Ingredients

Most of the formulas listed in this book call for readily available and affordable ingredients, many of which you might already have as standard grocery items. Otherwise, find the missing ingredients at your local grocery store, making sure to check the international foods section. Vitamin stores may carry a large selection of ingredients you could use, such as vegetable oils, essential oils, and soaps. Or you could place a small order online.

Try to make sure that they are natural, organic, and vegetable-derived, and try to validate the usage technique and recommended ratio in a formula. Most retailers have good customer support and reply to inquiries in a timely manner. Ask about the origin, the source, the purity, the extraction method, and any other question that you need an answer to.

It is always better to buy food-grade ingredients when available, because they are superior in quality to cosmetic-grade. This is especially true for oils, such as avocado, grape seed, almond, hazelnut,

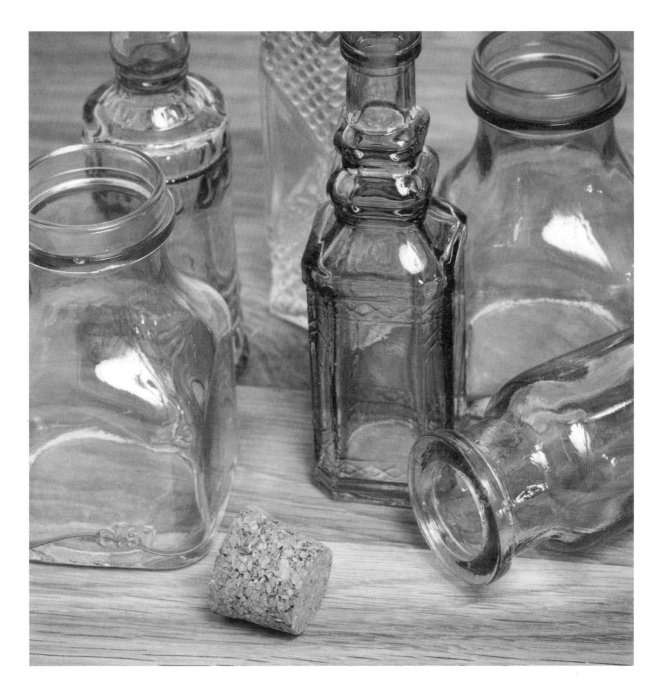

and olive oil. Extra virgin and cold-pressed oils are preferred, since their properties and benefits are not altered by heat and chemical processes. Needless to say, organic is preferred over conventional, because it does not carry pesticides.

Begin by buying a few of the oils that are most suitable for your skin type and expand later on. Thicker oils, such as olive and avocado oil, are recommended for dry and mature skin. Mature skin will also benefit from oils such as evening primrose, wheat germ, and pomegranate seed oil. Lighter oils, often referred to as dry oils, are more suitable for acne-prone and combination skin: Try jojoba or almond oil. Hazelnut oil is an astringent oil and is therefore a good choice for oily skin.

Glycerin is a long-known humectant (hygroscopic substance). It is widely used in the pharmaceutical industry and in cosmetics. This water-loving ingredient will help keep your skin moisturized and softened. Make sure you purchase vegetable glycerin.

Shea butter and beeswax are called for in cream and balm formulations.

Water is a common ingredient in almost all formulas. Purified or distilled water remains the best, because it does not carry chelating agents that might interact with other ingredients within the formula.

All formulas in this book call for natural ingredients. Most of them are vegan friendly. Beeswax, honey, eggs, and dairy products are among the non-vegan ingredients included in some formulas.

Storing Your Finished Products

One of the advantages of making your own cosmetics is the privilege of using them fresh, when nutrients are still intact and at their highest concentration; also, the preparation of small batches that will be used up in little time simplifies storage issues. Many formulas, especially those for facial masks, are for products to be used right away, and storing them simply does not apply. Others are anhydrous, and that lack of water protects them from spoilage. Storage is then simplified to avoiding direct light and heat. Creams and lotions, however, are prone to spoilage, and once your cream is made, you will need to pour it into a wisely chosen container and keep it in a spot that will maximize its shelf life. This is very easy when you keep in mind the following guidelines:

- For containers, glass is best. Also, the smaller the opening, the better. Two-ounce glass jars are an excellent choice. Try to get as close to the quantity you are making as possible. A smaller opening means less contact with the outside, which means less oxygen contact and a cleaner product for a longer time. Plastic containers sold in stores are convenient and lightweight, but plastic tends to release chemicals into the product. Tip: Washing your hands before reaching for your cream helps prevent germs from entering the product through your fingertips.

- Where to store your product? Less light and less heat mean longer shelf life. Go for amber glass when available. Closed cabinets are better than exposed shelves. Keep your products away from warm spots such as light bulbs, showers, and hot tubs.

- Refrigeration: How can you tell whether your product needs it? If you have used ingredients that needed refrigeration, such as milk or eggs, then your product should be refrigerated. Overall, by slowing down chemical reactions, refrigeration will extend the life of the product, whatever the formula. Most creams, lotions, and toners will store very well in a cool, shaded place—your medicine cabinet, for instance.

- Adding natural preservatives is also beneficial in protecting your products from spoilage. This can be done by adding the antioxidant vitamin E or a concoction of naturally derived preservatives, such as grape seed extract, rosemary oil extract, or others listed in this book (See page 52).

- Use your senses: If you notice that your beauty product has changed in color, texture, or smell, it is no longer good to use. If it has separated, grown mold, or lost its initial scent, most likely it is time to make a new one. Think of your formula as food for your skin; if you wouldn't eat it, don't rub it on.

CONVERSION CHART FOR METRIC AND U.S. SYSTEM UNITS

8 ounces = 1 cup

4 ounces = ½ cup

2 ounces = ¼ cup

1 tablespoon = 3 teaspoons

2 tablespoons = ⅛ cup

4 tablespoons = ¼ cup

2 tablespoons = 1 fluid ounce

1 teaspoon = 5 ml

1 tablespoon = 15 ml

1 pinch = ⅛ teaspoon or less

20 drops = 1 ml

10 drops = 0.5 ml

1 fluid ounce = 29.573 ml (30 ml)

1 cup = 236.6 ml (240 ml)

100 ml = 3.38 fluid ounces

1 gram = 0.0353 ounce

7 grams = ¼ ounce

113.4 grams = 4 ounces

454 grams = 1 pound

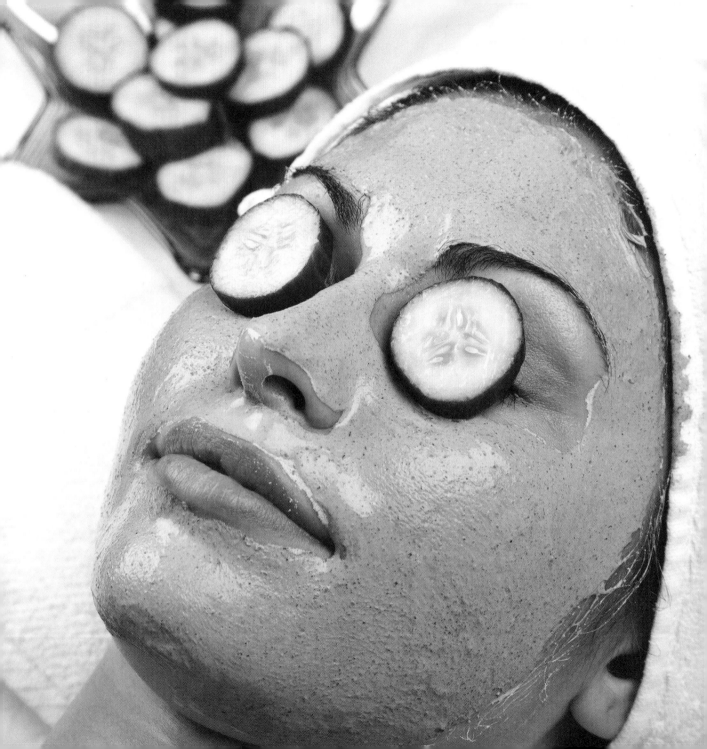

CHAPTER 5

Facial Masks and Scrubs

Facial masks are very easy to prepare and fun to apply on the face, neck, and décolletage area. Fruits and vegetables will always be among your key ingredients, because they can boost skin with vitamins, antioxidants, and minerals. Choose them ripe and tender for easy mashing and mixing.

Facial masks are the perfect place to start for beginners, because they are simple, and all you need to achieve is a pleasant texture you can work with. A good texture is usually smooth, with no visible lumps, and of an adequate thickness that will allow spreading with minimal dripping. Thickeners of choice will come right out of your pantry—for example, ground oats, almond meal, rice powder, cornstarch, cornmeal, and other such ingredients.

Because facial masks are often extemporaneous preparations, meaning they are to be used right away, you do not need to worry about preservation. Just mix the ingredients, apply the mix, and let your skin soak in the nutrients at the peak of their concentration. It is usually okay to refrigerate the leftovers if you plan to treat yourself to another mask during the same week, before the mixture starts to lose moisture and antioxidants.

If your preparation is a little runny, you might either use more thickener or simply spread it between double layers of gauze, like making a jam sandwich, and apply the gauze to your face. You may need to precut the double gauze in strips and circles to cover forehead, neck, and cheeks: four rectangles for the forehead and neck and four circles for the cheeks. Sitting in a recliner chair can help keep gauze pads in place.

Contact time for a mask is usually 10–15 minutes, and a silicone spatula can come in handy when it is time to remove your mask, before rinsing it off with lukewarm water.

Try to find time for a nutritional mask at least once a week (twice a week if you feel that your skin needs a little extra plumping or at the change of seasons).

Masks can also serve as a vehicle for facial scrubs. The addition of an exfoliating agent transforms a mask into a two-in-one mask and scrub. Examples of exfoliating agents are almond meal, semolina, rice beads, and clay, among others.

Coco-Belle Scrub

This mask combines the benefits of coconut, royal jelly, and almond milk to moisturize and nourish your skin. Shredded coconut flakes make a wonderful base for mature-skin facial masks and scrubs because they act as a double agent: Through rubbing, impurities and dead skin cells are eliminated; simultaneously, coconut oil is released and absorbed through the superficial epithelial cells without leaving behind an oily residue. Coconut oil can deeply nourish challenged skin, help improve dryness, and fight wrinkles.

Look for unsweetened, sulfite-free coconut flakes, or simply make your own using a cheese grater. Freshly shredded coconut has a higher moisture content, and freshly released oil is still unoxidized—just make sure there are no abrasive particles in your coconut shreds.

Royal jelly is an extremely rich super food that is designed to feed the queen bee, which can lay over two thousand eggs a day. It is often sold blended with honey. Adding a little to your facial mask can make it highly nourishing for your skin. A little almond milk provides a good dose of vitamin E, which is a wrinkle-fighting antioxidant, and vanilla flavored milk will add a pleasant aroma to the mixture. Together, those ingredients will bring moisture, lipids, and vitamins to revive dry, wrinkled skin.

Make this mask twice a week to quickly improve skin smoothness and nourish skin. No oils are added to this formula, which makes it a suitable recipe for all skin types, including oily skin.

INGREDIENTS

3 tablespoons thinly shredded coconut

1 tablespoon royal jelly

1 tablespoon vanilla-flavored almond milk

INSTRUCTIONS

1. Mix coconut shreds with royal jelly or honey.

2. Add almond milk to the mixture to achieve a pleasant and desirable texture. Then spread on cleansed face and neck and wait for your skin to soak in the nutrients of this mask for 15 minutes.

3. Rinse with chlorine-free water and pat your face dry with a towel.

Yeast-Based Anti-Aging Facial Mask

Yeast is a single-cell organism loaded with nutrients essential for its survival and superfast proliferation. With the help of the remaining ingredients in this formula, such as milk and honey, this mask will act as a youth booster for your skin.

Because of its higher fat content, whole milk brings more softness to your skin than skim milk, because the saturated fats in whole milk will help lock in skin moisture. Honey is a proven emollient, which draws moisture to the skin, and has established anti-aging properties.

Rice and rice derivatives are gaining popularity in the cosmetics industry for all the benefits they can offer. Rice flour will help give the mask some elasticity for easier spreading and will also allow scrubbing and removal of dead skin cells and impurities.

Although not essential to the formula, a few drops of vanilla will add a nice, pleasant smell.

Make this mask once or twice a week for a month to plump skin and restore its glow.

INGREDIENTS

2 ounces (60 ml) whole organic milk

1 small packet dry active yeast

1 tablespoon honey

3–5 drops vanilla extract (optional)

3 tablespoons rice flour

Note: Almond milk can be used instead of whole milk as a vegan alternative, but the creaminess of the preparation will not be the same.

INSTRUCTIONS

1. Start by warming milk in the microwave or in a pan, making sure not to overheat it.

2. Sprinkle the content of the yeast packet over the warmed milk and mix with a fork.

3. Add honey and vanilla extract and mix again. The warm milk will help dissolve the honey and will aid in the yeast proliferation. Dip a cotton ball into the mixture and apply to the face and neck.

4. Add rice flour to the remaining mix, 1 tablespoon at a time, stirring well, until mixture thickens.

5. You can now apply another thicker coat on the face and neck and allow the mask to dry over 15 minutes.

6. Scrub with your fingers (over the sink) to remove the brittle mask. Finish by washing your face with warm water, and follow with a facial cream.

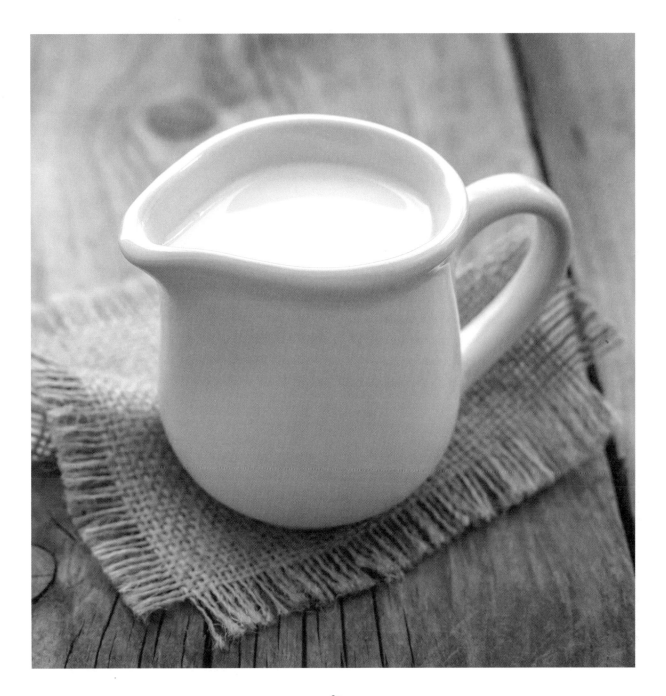

Brightening Apple Mask

This mask relies on the wonderful effects of fruits and is recommended for skin with blemishes or sunspots to reverse sun damage, especially at the end of the summer season. Apples are rich in vitamin C, which is a documented skin-brightening agent. Citrus fruits are also supreme sources of ascorbic acid (vitamin C). When combined with cranberry seed oil, which is high in sun-protective antioxidants, these ingredients will reverse time on challenged skin.

Make this mask twice a week, for two or three weeks to unify skin tone, and always follow with sunscreen.

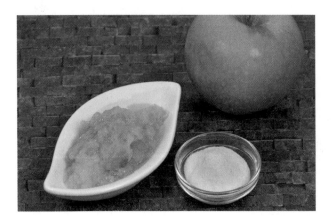

INGREDIENTS

gauze strips

1 freshly grated peeled green apple

1 teaspoon vegetable glycerin

½ teaspoon lemon juice

½ teaspoon cranberry seed oil

1–2 tablespoons rice flour

Note: Honey can be used instead of glycerin.

INSTRUCTIONS

1. Prepare gauze strips by laying gauze in double layers and cutting four rectangles for the forehead and neck and four circles for the cheeks.

2. Mix the above ingredients, adding as much rice flour as needed to prevent dripping. Then spread the mix like sandwich filling between double gauze layers and apply to your forehead, neck, and cheeks.

3. Sit in a reclining chair and wait for 10 minutes before removing the gauze strips and rinsing your face with lukewarm water.

4. If bothersome tingling occurs, rinse immediately.

5. Always follow with a high-SPF (30 or more) sunscreen to avoid vitamin C–induced photosensitivity.

Exfoliating Mask

This is a very easy mask in which ground oats do a double job: They soften the skin and exfoliate it at the same time. This formula is suitable for all skin types, especially dry skin. It relies on almond oil, which is a great source of vitamin E, as well as whole milk as a source of fat, which will help lock in skin moisture. The addition of vitamins will empower this mask and take its efficacy to a whole new level, making it greatly nourishing while boosting its anti-wrinkle potency.

INGREDIENTS

1 teaspoon almond oil

3 tablespoons ground oats

3 ounces (or 100 ml) whole milk

10 drops (0.5 ml) vitamin E

10 drops (0.5 ml) vitamin B5 (optional)

1 capsule coenzyme Q10 (optional)

INSTRUCTIONS

1. Drizzle almond oil over the ground oats, then add milk gradually until you achieve a paste-like texture.

2. Use a dropper to add vitamins E and B5. Then open the capsule and empty the coenzyme Q10 content, sprinkling it over the mixture. Mix well to distribute the vitamins within the mask.

3. Make sure your face and neck are clean and makeup free. Coat your forehead, cheeks, and neck with this mix, making sure to avoid the eye area. Relax and allow 20 minutes contact time.

4. Remove by rubbing away all the mix with your hands and washing your face with warm water; then pat your face dry with a towel.

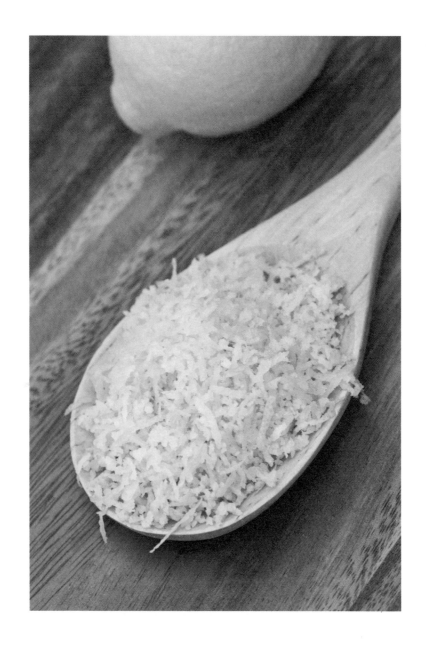

Brighter Complexion Mask

This mask combines the skin-brightening effects of vitamin C with the sun damage-reversing properties of avocado.

Use at the change of seasons, when sun exposure is low, to improve the appearance of sunspots. Vitamin C is a skin rejuvenator that will help plump the skin, and avocado is extremely rich in nourishing polyunsaturated fatty acids, which makes this formula highly beneficial for both mature and dry skin.

INGREDIENTS

gauze strips
½ ripe white peach
½ ripe avocado
½ teaspoon lemon zest
½ teaspoon lemon juice
1 teaspoon ground oats

INSTRUCTIONS

1. Begin preparing your gauze strips by laying the gauze in double layers and cutting four rectangles for the forehead and neck and four circles for the cheeks.

2. Mash the peach and the avocado together with a fork. Add the lemon zest and lemon juice and mix well. Sprinkle and blend in ground oats as needed to reduce dripping.

3. Then spread on the precut double layers of gauze and place the gauze strips over forehead, cheeks, and neck. It is also okay to spread the mixture directly on the skin; just make sure to avoid the eye area.

4. Leave the mask on for 15 minutes, unless bothersome tingling occurs. Remove the gauze pads and rinse abundantly with warm water.

5. Finally, pat the face dry with a face towel, and always follow with a moisturizer and a high-SPF sunscreen, even during winter.

6. Repeat on a weekly basis, over a month, for best results.

Brightening and Exfoliating 2-in-1 Mask

This wholesome formula is engineered with multiple skin needs in mind. While its brightening powers are provided by lemon juice, which boosts skin with vitamin C, almond meal acts as a mild exfoliator, to reveal newer and brighter skin. Olive oil and glycerin confer softness and moisture, alongside royal jelly, which takes skin nourishment to a whole new level. This is why the results of this tone unifying mask are impressive, especially when used twice weekly for a month.

INGREDIENTS

1 teaspoon lemon juice

2 tablespoons almond meal

1 tablespoon royal jelly

½ teaspoon olive oil

20 drops (1 ml) vegetable glycerin

INSTRUCTIONS

1. Drizzle lemon juice over almond meal and mix with a fork. Add remaining ingredients one at a time and mix.

2. Then spread an amount equivalent to about 1 tablespoon over a clean face. Wait for 5 minutes; then scrub and rinse off. Repeat a few days later with the refrigerated leftovers or a freshly made mask.

3. Because this formula might increase your skin's photosensitivity, avoid sun exposure and always follow with a daily sunblock.

All-Almond Mask

This recipe is for almond lovers, a strictly vegan formula, gently exfoliating and extremely nourishing for the skin. While almond oil supplements skin with generous amounts of vitamin E and unsaturated fatty acids, almond meal is a soft scrubbing agent that will take away dead skin cells and regenerate skin. This recipe is for all skin types, any season of the year. When prepared regularly, it helps keep skin nourished, soft, and refreshed. It also has some anti-aging benefits. Do not use almond-derived ingredients if there are allergy concerns.

INGREDIENTS

½ cup almond meal
2 ounces (60 ml) almond milk
½ teaspoon almond oil
3 drops almond extract

INSTRUCTIONS

1. Mix together all of the above ingredients, using as much almond milk as needed to obtain a paste-like texture that is easy to spread but not too runny.

2. Use your fingertips or a silicone spatula to spread the mixture over your face and neck.

3. Leave the mask on until it becomes brittle.

4. Rub gently to remove dead skin cells and impurities. Wash your face if you feel like it; otherwise, this mask comes off easily and leaves no residue.

Honey Almond Mask

Honey and almond have become a rather famous "duo" featured in numerous hair and skin formulations. While almonds are rich in antioxidant vitamin E and polyunsaturated fatty acids, honey is a great skin moisturizer, and its anti-aging properties make the two a wonderful combination. With little oil content, if any, this formula is suitable for all skin types, including oily skin. The addition of wheat germ oil boosts the anti-aging properties of this formula for optimal results.

INGREDIENTS

2 ounces (60 ml) almond milk

1 teaspoon honey

½ cup almond meal

5 drops vanilla extract

20 drops (1 ml) wheat germ oil (optional)

INSTRUCTIONS

1. Mix honey with almond milk until dissolved, then add it to almond meal and mix. Add remaining ingredients and mix until a paste-like texture is obtained.

2. Spread with fingertips or silicone spatula on face and neck. Sit back and relax.

3. Remove in 15 minutes or when dry and brittle. Rinse if necessary.

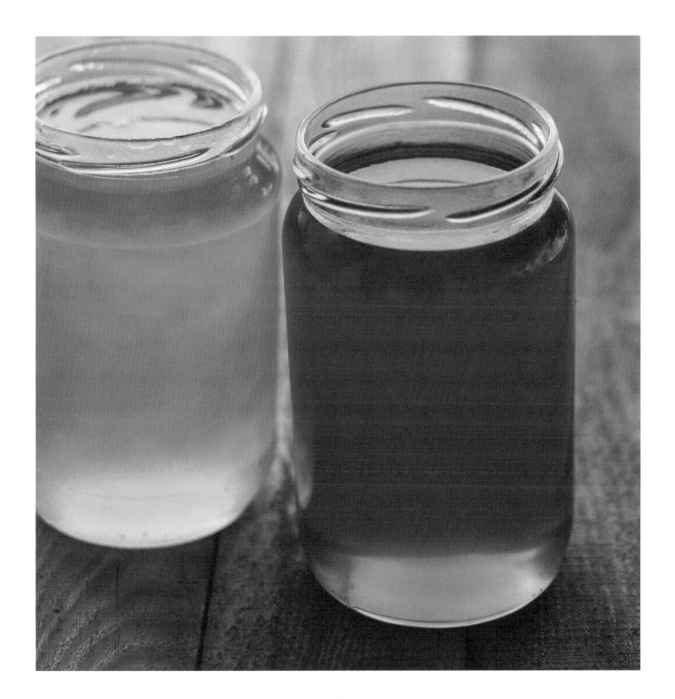

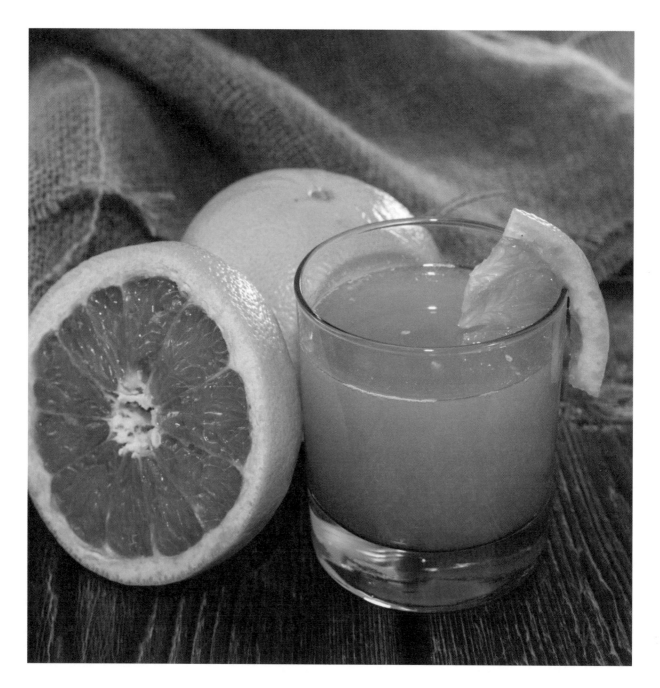

Winter Rescue Mask

Weather aggression is always noticeable, not only on hands, legs, and lips, but also on the face. This mask contains full-fat cream cheese, which will restore some of the skin's lipid mantle and help protect skin against weather-induced dryness.

The remaining ingredients will boost skin's vitality and revive it. While wheat germ oil is extremely nourishing, moisturizing, and anti-aging, grapefruit juice will load your skin with antioxidants and vitamin C for a refreshed and younger-looking skin. Adding egg white is optional but strongly recommended if you wish to have proteins in your mask, as well. Prepare this formula when your skin feels dry and tight, or routinely during winter and harsh weather months.

INGREDIENTS

2 ounces (60 ml) full-fat cream cheese (softened; see below)

½ teaspoon honey

20 drops (1 ml) wheat germ oil

20 drops (1 ml) grapefruit juice

1 egg white (optional)

gauze strips (optional)

INSTRUCTIONS

1. Allow the cheese to soften at room temperature—do not microwave. Flatten with a fork, and then add remaining ingredients one at a time while mixing with the fork.

2. Spread with a spatula on clean face and neck, directly or between double layers of precut gauze strips. (Prepare the gauze strips ahead of time by laying gauze in double layers and cutting four rectangles for the forehead and neck and four circles for the cheeks.)

3. Lie back or sit in a reclining chair and wait 15–20 minutes before removing gauze pads and rinsing off.

4. Repeat this mask on a weekly basis to sustain results and protect the skin. Follow with the application of daily moisturizer and a sunblock.

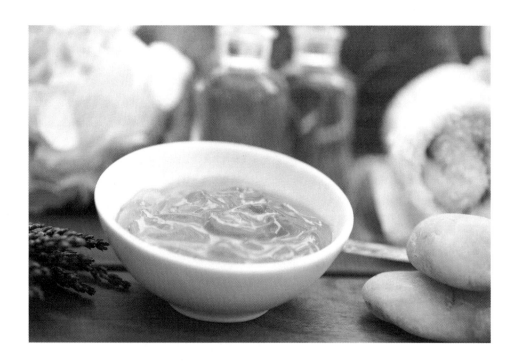

Ah! Cooling Gel

This mask is a great choice for sensitive skin suffering from irritation. It relies on the anti-inflammatory properties of rosemary to ease redness and soothe the skin. Mint is also another contributor to the effect of this recipe, because it contains menthol, which will provide an instant cooling effect and potentiate the efficacy of rosemary. Cucumber juice is a skin-friendly ingredient that will moisturize in a very soft way, and its effects are complemented by glycerin, which acts as an emollient, bringing more moisture to the skin.

INGREDIENTS

- 1 teaspoon rosemary (preferably fresh)
- 5 leaves fresh mint (chopped)
- 1 cup boiling water
- 1 ounce (30 ml) cucumber juice
- 1 teaspoon vegetable glycerin
- ½ teaspoon xanthan gum

INSTRUCTIONS

1. Start by preparing a decoction of rosemary and mint by adding them to the boiling water. Wait 3–5 minutes before turning off the heat.

2. Filter and set aside for a few minutes before adding cucumber juice and glycerin. Stir well to mix.

3. While the decoction is still warm, sprinkle gradual amounts of xanthan gum on the surface and whisk until a gel starts to form. Using an electric whisk is helpful in avoiding lumps, but be careful not to splatter. Keep in mind that using too much gum can transform the mixture into an unpleasant stringy gel.

4. Set aside to cool; then transfer to a pump bottle and refrigerate.

5. Apply two to three pumps to the face and neck, without rubbing. Then wipe off with a cotton ball or rinse with plenty of lukewarm water. To avoid friction and minimize irritation, finish by patting your face dry with a towel.

6. This gel can be used as often as needed to soothe irritated skin.

AHA-Rich Peeling Mask

Alpha hydroxy acids, often known as AHA, are acidic components used in many over-the-counter products, as well as professional products that serve as a chemical peel for the skin. They may be irritating and can cause redness and photosensitivity, which is why many people avoid professional peeling. This mask is a gentler alternative, which relies on lactic acid, an AHA found in sour milk, yogurt, and kefir. The acidity of this formula is attenuated with aloe vera gel and honey, so it can be better tolerated than a chemical peel. It is still recommended, however, to do a patch test on a small area before applying this mask to the face. Always avoid contact with eyes, and do not apply to open cuts and wounds or on irritated skin. This formula works best at the end of summer to improve dull skin appearance and unify skin tone.

INGREDIENTS

1 tablespoon full-fat plain yogurt
1 tablespoon aloe vera gel
1 tablespoon honey
1 tablespoon ground oats

INSTRUCTIONS

1. Mix the above ingredients in a small bowl and then apply to the face, always avoiding the eyes. Leave on for 10 minutes before rinsing with lukewarm water.

2. Follow with a moisturizer and a high-SPF sunscreen.

3. Repeat on a weekly basis for three to four weeks for more obvious results.

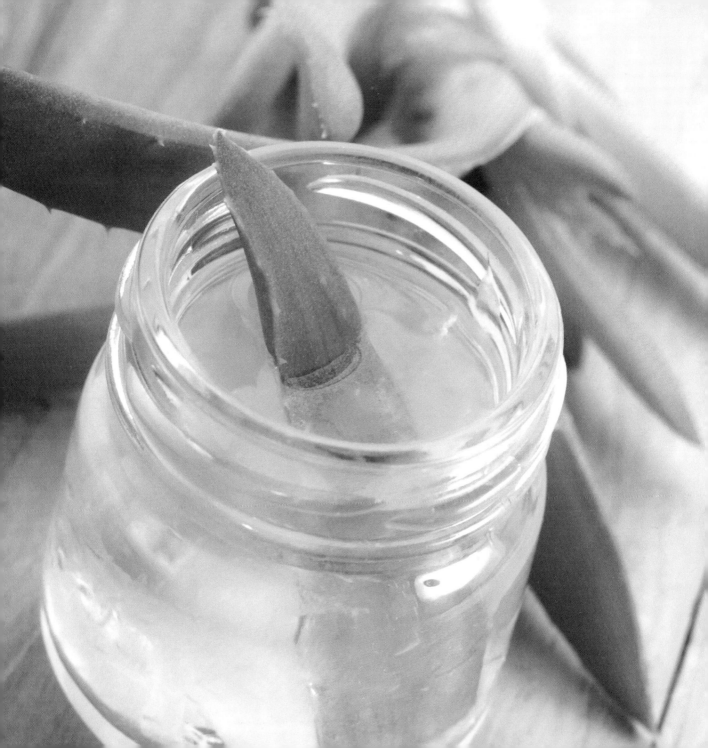

Astringent Mask

This formula is for oily skin:
Make this mask when your skin
is misbehaving, and you need to
tame the breakouts. Just like green tea,
hazelnut oil is astringent and reduces pore size,
which is why it is a great choice for acne-prone
skin. Of course, avoid the use of nut oils in case
of a nut allergy.

INGREDIENTS

1 teaspoon cornstarch

2 ounces (60 ml) freshly made green tea infusion

½ teaspoon hazelnut oil

3 ounces witch hazel or neroli water

INSTRUCTIONS

1. Sprinkle the cornstarch, gradually, on the green tea while it is still hot, and whisk vigorously. When the tea starts to thicken, add the oil, continuing to whisk.

2. Refrigerate the preparation for further thickening and to decrease its temperature prior to applying.

3. When cool, apply the gel to the face, avoiding the eyes. Leave on for 15 minutes before rinsing off with water. Do not rub skin excessively, as that might stimulate the sebaceous glands and lead to excessive oily secretions.

4. Finish with a cotton ball soaked with witch hazel or neroli water for some extra astringency.

Walnut Anti-Aging Mask

Walnuts are rich in omega-3 essential fatty acids and antioxidants and have become popular ingredients in numerous anti-aging creams. This mask will bring a great amount of nutrients for tired, mature, and sun-damaged skin. Although it is particularly recommended for dry and combination skin, it is also suitable for oily skin. Prepare regularly to boost your skin's omega-3 levels and keep it looking healthy.

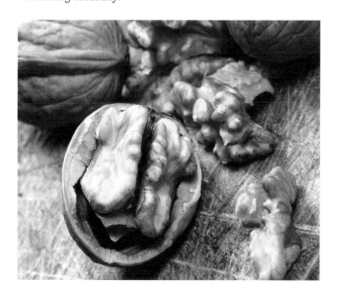

INGREDIENTS

½ cup walnut halves

1 tablespoon honey

1 tablespoon almond milk

Note: Flax seeds are also high in omega-3 and make a valid substitution for walnuts in this formula, especially in case of a nut allergy.

INSTRUCTIONS

1. Try to buy in-the-shell walnuts and use a nut cracker or a hammer to crack them open. They have a higher moisture level and preserved omega-3s. Just make sure there are no shell particles in your walnuts.

2. A food processor will help you pulverize them and achieve a very fine texture that is not abrasive. Use the powder as soon as it is prepared, when it has the highest moisture content and before oils begin oxidation.

3. Pour the powder into a bowl, make a well in the center, add the honey and almond milk, and mix thoroughly.

4. Apply to the face and neck. Leave on for 15 minutes; then rinse the mask off with fresh water. Follow with your regular facial moisturizer.

Egg White Skin-Firming Mask

Egg whites are a smart addition to your facial mask when you seek a skin-tightening effect, because it is a great quality protein that will support collagen. Combined with glycerin and yogurt, this formula will surely improve skin feel and tone. Yogurt is acidic and will act as an exfoliating agent, assisting with skin cell renewal.

INGREDIENTS

1 egg white

Zest of ¼ lemon

½ teaspoon vegetable glycerin

1 tablespoon yogurt

1 tablespoon ground oats

INSTRUCTIONS

1. Prepare this mix immediately prior to application. Using a whisk, mix the egg white with the lemon zest (to neutralize the egg's smell), then add the glycerin and yogurt and whisk until homogenous.

2. Gradually, sprinkle with the ground oats and mix well.

3. Apply to a clean face and neck, avoiding the eye area. Wait 10–15 minutes before rinsing off with tepid water. Follow with your moisturizer and a daytime sunscreen.

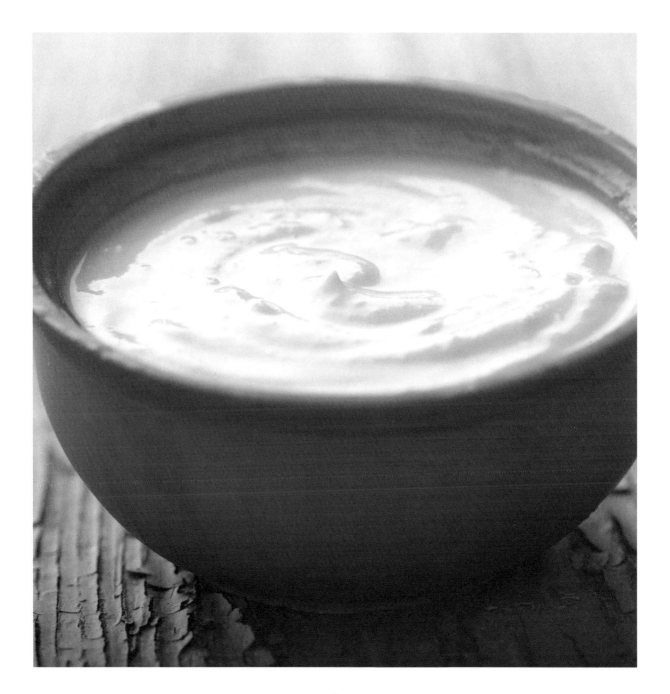

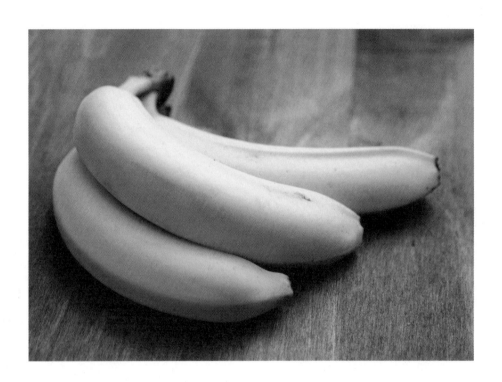

Fruity Mask

Sometimes skin needs a surge of vitamins, antioxidants, and minerals to wipe away its dullness and restore its natural defenses.

Ripe fruits make a great facial mask component, whether used alone or in a cocktail blend. This mask is rich in antioxidants, vitamin C, potassium, and other nutrients that will work together to improve complexion and give it a healthier look. Prepare more often in summer and at the change of seasons. This formula suits most skin types. People with sensitive skin are always advised to patch-test recipes before applying on a larger skin surface.

INGREDIENTS

½ ripe white peach
½ ripe banana
¼ ripe pear
10 drops (0.5 ml) lemon juice
1–2 tablespoons ground oats
gauze strips (optional)

INSTRUCTIONS

1. Dice the fruits and puree them with a stick blender or a food processor. Add lemon juice to prevent discoloration.

2. Sprinkle with enough ground oats to thicken the mix and facilitate application.

3. Spread directly over a clean face and neck, or between precut double gauze layers, avoiding the eye area. (Prepare gauze strips ahead of time by laying gauze in double layers and cutting four rectangles for the forehead and neck and four circles for the cheeks.)

4. Sit in a recliner chair and wait 15 minutes before rinsing. Follow with your regular moisturizer and sunscreen.

Brightening Veggie Mask

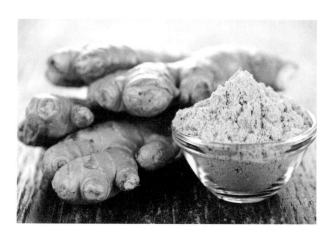

INGREDIENTS

1 cup boiled and drained potato, diced

½ teaspoon lemon juice

1 teaspoon finely chopped parsley leaves

Pinch finely grated ginger

2 ounces (60 ml) aloe vera gel

INSTRUCTIONS

1. Mash the potatoes very well, avoiding lumps. Add the lemon juice, parsley, and grated ginger; then mix. Gradually, fold in the aloe vera gel and mix thoroughly until evenly distributed.

2. Spread on clean skin, face and neck, avoiding the eye area.

3. Wash after 15 minutes unless tingling or other unpleasant skin reaction occurs. Follow with a moisturizer and sunscreen.

Just like fruit, vegetables can also be loaded with vitamins, minerals, and antioxidants that will improve skin appearance and nourish it.

Potatoes are known skin brighteners, as is parsley, which is rich in antioxidants and vitamin C. Ginger improves microcirculation, which takes away toxins and brings in essential nutrients for epithelial cells. Adding a touch of aloe vera is always a good moisturizing step.

Healthy Glow Mask

As well as being highly moisturizing, this formula improves skin glow by providing vitamin A precursors, as well as vitamin E and other antioxidants. It calls for carrot seed oil, which is rich in carotenoids, precursors of vitamin A that are capable of giving a healthy glow to tired skin, as well as for rice bran oil, which is rich in antioxidants, such as the anti-aging vitamin E. And because skin moisture is important, a little glycerin or honey is added.

Unless you are pregnant, it is also recommended to drink a cup of carrot juice daily over a week to boost skin glow. (Excessive amounts of vitamin A might pose a risk of fetal harm, so pregnant women should consult with their physician prior to ingesting considerable amounts of carrot juice.)

INGREDIENTS

1 teaspoon carrot seed oil
1 teaspoon rice bran oil
1 ounce (30 ml) pureed cucumber
1 teaspoon vegetable glycerin or honey
1 tablespoon ground oats

INSTRUCTIONS

1. Mix the oils and add 2 tablespoons of pureed cucumber; add the glycerin or honey. Sprinkle with the ground oats and whisk vigorously. Add oatmeal as needed to increase the thickness of the mask to your preference and prevent dripping.

2. Use immediately after preparing, while nutrients are at their peak. Spread on a clean face and neck.

3. Leave on for 15 minutes, and then wash with warm water. Always follow with a daily moisturizer.

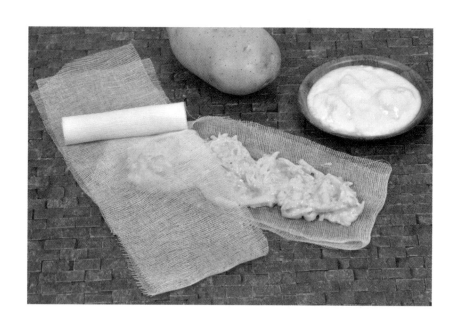

Snow White Mask

This formula earned its name for two reasons: It is made with only white ingredients, and it has a skin-whitening effect.

Yogurt contains lactic acid, which exfoliates and brightens the skin. Potato is also a skin brightener, sometimes referred to as a skin-bleaching agent, and it contains enzymes and vitamins that contribute to this effect. Together with lemon juice, this formula is a powerful skin transformer.

INGREDIENTS

20 drops (1 ml) lemon juice
1 small potato, finely grated
1 ounce (30 ml) plain full-fat yogurt
1 tablespoon ground oats
gauze strips

INSTRUCTIONS

1. Begin by adding the lemon juice to the grated potato. Then add the yogurt and thicken with the ground oats. Combine all ingredients well, using a fork.

2. Prepare gauze strips by laying gauze in double layers and cutting four rectangles for the forehead and neck and four circles for the cheeks.

3. Spread a thick amount of the mixture between double layers of the gauze.

4. Sit in a reclining chair and apply the gauze pads to cheeks, forehead, and neck. Leave the mask on for 15 minutes before taking gauze pads off and rinsing with plenty of water. (If bothersome tingling occurs, or if you notice redness or other signs of skin reaction, rinse immediately with plenty of water.) Always follow with sunscreen (SPF 30).

5. Repeat weekly for a month for best results. This mask can also be used on the hands to decrease the appearance of age spots.

Cucumber Mask

This skin-friendly mask is highly moisturizing, greatly refreshing, and suitable for all skin types, even most sensitive ones. Make it during summer's hottest months to replenish some of the skin's lost nutrients. The addition of highly nutritious royal jelly takes this formula to a whole other level.

INGREDIENTS

⅓ English cucumber plus 2 slices for the eyes

1 teaspoon royal jelly

2 tablespoons ground oats

INSTRUCTIONS

1. Precut the cucumber, then puree with a stick blender. Add the royal jelly, mix, and then gradually add the oatmeal, mixing continuously to achieve a paste-like texture.

2. Spread the mask on a clean face and neck, then lie back and place the cucumber slices on your eyelids, flipping them over halfway through the 15 minutes of waiting time.

3. Rinse off the mask with lukewarm water and follow with your daily moisturizer.

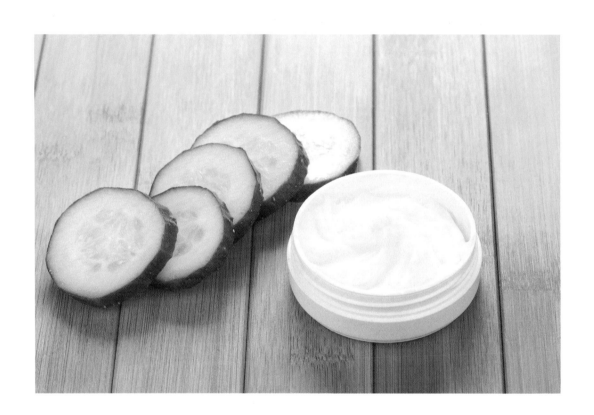

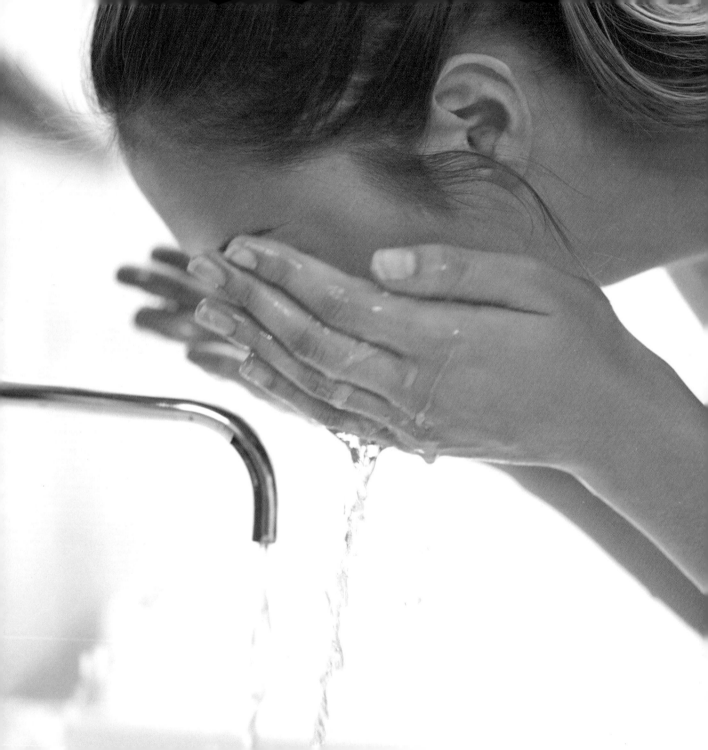

CHAPTER 6

Cleansers and Makeup Removers

Cleaning our skin is, for most of us, a crucial step of our daily beauty routine. We often clean our skin twice a day, to eliminate dust and toxins in the morning and makeup in the evening. Cleansing also prepares the skin to better receive a subsequent toner, moisturizer, or night cream.

Different types of cleansers are available to suit all needs and preferences. While some people prefer to wash their face with a soapy cleanser and water, those with more sensitive skin might choose a soap-free formula. Milky cleansers are always a favorite of people with dry skin, because their creaminess counteracts the drying effects of soap. Oily cleansers are highly appreciated when waterproof makeup needs removal; just make sure to follow with a toner to wash away oily residue.

A cleanser can be a scrub, as well. Just add some "beads" to the formulation to get a two-in-one cleanser and scrub. The beads could be ground oats, almond meal, semolina, clay, or other slightly coarse components.

Multiple formulas are offered in this chapter; choose your favorites according to your preferences and your skin type.

Customizable Foaming Cleanser

Some people love the cleaning effect of soap. Castile soap, which originated from the Castile region in Spain, is a concentrated vegetable soap traditionally made with olive oil. It can be diluted with water or hydrosol in various proportions, depending on its intended use. And because all kinds of soaps, even natural ones, are still harsh, as they wash away surface oils, this formula incorporates aloe vera juice and glycerin to counteract the drying effect. Using a hydrosol will produce a fragrant cleanser: Go for a rose or geranium scent, which blends well with lavender, if lavender castile soap is being used.

NOTE

If you have acne-prone skin, use witch hazel instead of rose hydrosol for astringency. To give your cleanser exfoliating properties, make a paste with 1 tablespoon of almond meal and the glycerin in the formula, then add to the hydrosol and aloe vera juice and whisk. Proceed as indicated for the remainder of the preparation, whisking thoroughly to ensure even distribution of the suspended particles.

INGREDIENTS

- 1 teaspoon vegetable glycerin
- 1 ounce (30 ml) hydrosol of your choice (such as geranium or rose)
- 1 ounce (30 ml) aloe vera juice
- 1 ounce (30 ml) liquid soap such as castile soap

INSTRUCTIONS

1. Add the glycerin to the hydrosol and aloe vera juice, and stir well. Add the mixture to the soap, in a very thin stream, while whisking continuously and gently to avoid excessive foaming. Do not use a stick blender.

2. Allow the product to settle before transferring it to a pump bottle.

3. Shake briefly and abruptly before pumping. Wet your face; then pump once or twice into your hands and rub over the face and neck until the cleanser is nice and foamy.

4. Rinse off with warm or cold water; then pat your face dry with a towel.

Honey Sweet Cleanser

Castile soap is an excellent natural soap, but it can be harsh on sensitive skin. If you are a strict soap and water lover, you do not need to sacrifice that part of your daily routine, because the honey and glycerin in this formula will yield a softer cleanser that will not strip your skin of moisture or irritate it. This is a concentrated soap formula with a generous amount of glycerin to ensure that skin moisture is retained.

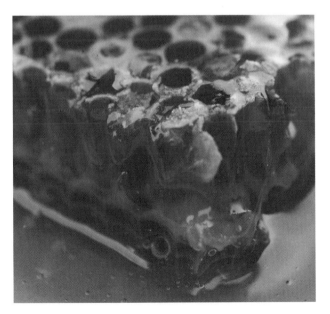

INGREDIENTS

1 tablespoon honey

1 ounce (30 ml) vegetable glycerin

2 ounces (60 ml) castile soap

5 drops lavender essential oil or other essential oil of your choice

INSTRUCTIONS

1. Place a small bowl in a pot filled with hot water. Add the honey, then glycerin, and whisk together. Remove the bowl from the water and place another one containing the castile soap. Pour the honey-glycerin mix into the soap while whisking.

2. Allow to cool to room temperature before transferring it to a pump bottle.

3. Wet your face and neck. Pump a small amount of soap (1-2 pumps at most) into your hands; rub your wet hands together to dilute the soap prior to massaging your face and neck.

4. Wipe off with a cotton ball, then rinse off with plenty of water, and pat your face dry with a towel. Follow with a moisturizer.

Light Cleansing Oil

This formula is for dry skin. It's a cleansing oil that will not leave behind a bothersome thick oily residue. It will nourish and soften skin while powerfully removing all makeup and impurities. Rosehip oil is very rich in antioxidants, and adding it to your oil will make a wonderful, light anti-aging oil.

INGREDIENTS

2 ounces (60 ml) almond or sunflower oil

2 teaspoons rosehip oil

5 drops geranium essential oil or other essential oil of your choice

INSTRUCTIONS

1. Mix the almond and rosehip oils well and transfer to an amber glass bottle with a dropper. Add the essential oil, place the dropper on, and shake well.

2. Moisten your face and then spread one drop on the forehead, one drop on each cheek, and one drop on the chin and neck. Massage gently, then wipe off with a cotton disk. Rinse off with water if desired or follow with a toner.

3. Use every night at bedtime.

4. To store, make sure the bottle is tightly closed and kept in a cool place away from heat, light, and moisture. This mixture can be stored through the shelf life of each individual ingredient.

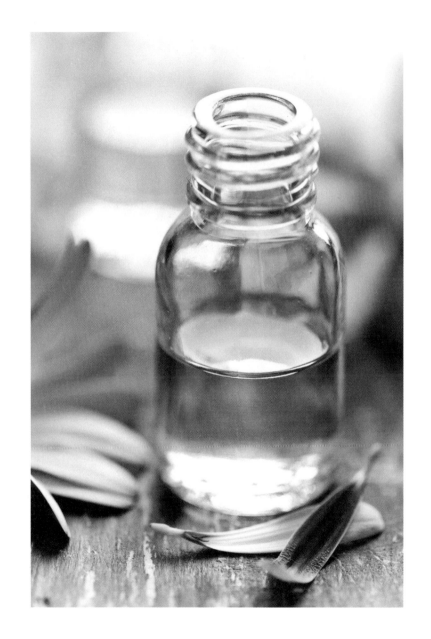

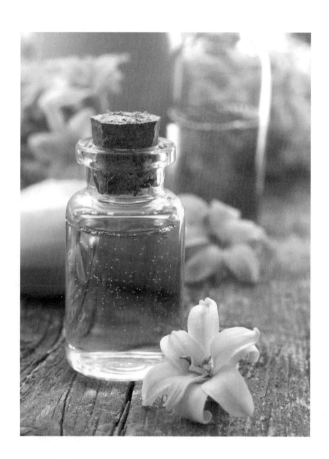

Exfoliating Cleansing Gel

A cleansing gel is always refreshing because of its high water content. In the following formula, xanthan gum will thicken the water phase and hold suspended particles in place. This cleanser is soap free and is a very good choice for sensitive, soap-intolerant skin. The efficacy of this gel is made complete with the addition of vitamin B5, which helps moisturize and nurture the skin.

INGREDIENTS

½ cup rose water

1 teaspoon exfoliating agent of your choice (for example, semolina, ground oats, almond meal)

10 drops (0.5 ml) vitamin B5

¼ teaspoon xanthan gum

5 drops of your favorite essential oil (such as gardenia or geranium)

INSTRUCTIONS

1. Begin by warming the rose water in a double boiler, until it reaches 100°F. Test this with a candy thermometer, then turn off the heat.

2. Sprinkle in the exfoliating agent gradually while whisking, add the B5, then sprinkle the xanthan gum in tiny amounts as you watch your mixture thicken. Keep in mind that too much xanthan gum can ruin the texture. Expect further spontaneous thickening, as well.

3. Add the essential oil and whisk vigorously to make sure your gel is evenly mixed.

4. Finish by transferring the mixture to a bottle and refrigerate it for 45 minutes to an hour for further thickening.

5. It is not necessary to wet your face and neck before applying the gel. Just massage a quarter-size amount onto your face and neck, then scrub gently and wipe away with a cotton disk.

6. Rinse well and pat your face dry with a towel.

Skin-Brightening Soapy Cleanser

This combination of exfoliating beads and lemon juice will take your usual morning cleanser to a new level. This formula is recommended for soap-tolerant skin, when a brightening effect is needed, especially after a sunny summer, to unify skin tone.

INGREDIENTS

- 2 teaspoons fresh, pulp-free lemon juice
- 1 ounce (30 ml) distilled water
- 1 ounce (30 ml) liquid castile soap
- 1 teaspoon ground oats
- 5 drops flowery essential oil of your choice, such as grapefruit essential oil

INSTRUCTIONS

1. Dilute the lemon juice with the indicated amount of distilled water. Slowly pour the diluted juice in a thin stream into the liquid soap, stirring gently and continuously.

2. Sprinkle the ground oats gradually into the mixture, whisking gently, until completely dispersed within the liquid. Last, add your essential oil, stir, and transfer the mixture to a pump bottle.

3. In the evening, shake the mixture well and generously wet your face before rubbing a dab between your wet palms and then over your face and neck. Always avoid the eyes.

4. Rinse with plenty of water.

5. Follow with a moisturizer—and do not forget your sunscreen in the morning.

Creamy Cleanser

In this formula, the addition of a moisturizing cream counteracts the drying effect of soap. The result is a smooth and creamy formula, perfect if you have dry skin and do not want to give up on soap.

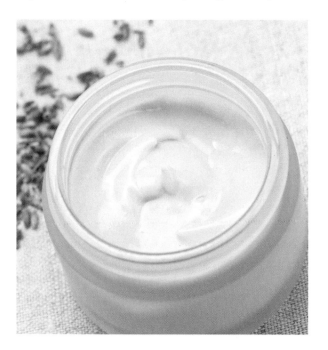

INGREDIENTS

2 ounces (60 ml) moisturizing cream

½ cup liquid castile soap

1 ounce (30 ml) rose water or lavender hydrosols

INSTRUCTIONS

1. In a double boiler, warm the cream, then add liquid soap in a thin stream, stirring gently and continuously. Turn off the heat and add the rose water in the same manner. Transfer to a jar or pump bottle and set aside to cool completely.

2. Massage a small amount of the cleanser onto your wet face and neck. Wipe off with a makeup sponge or cotton disk to remove makeup and grime. Rinse with plenty of water and pat your face dry with a towel. Follow with a moisturizer.

Waterproof Makeup Remover

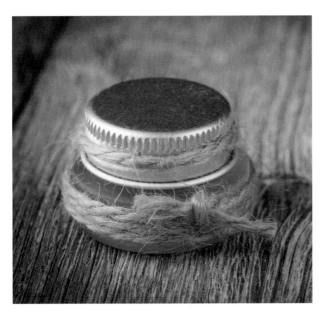

INGREDIENTS

1 tablespoon shea butter

1 ounce (30 ml) extra virgin coconut oil

1 tablespoon almond oil

10 drops (0.5 ml) vitamin E oil

INSTRUCTIONS

1. Melt the shea butter in a double boiler. Then add the remaining ingredients one at a time, finishing with the vitamin E.

2. Pour the mixture slowly into a small glass jar and allow it to cool to room temperature before putting on the lid.

3. Moistening your face before application helps decrease the greasy feel of this mixture. Spread a pea-size amount on each cheek and on the forehead. Then wipe off with a makeup sponge. Rinse well with warm water and finish with a toner that will take away any residual oily feeling.

This formula is for heavy makeup days only, when stubborn makeup is hard to remove and a powerful, oily cleanser is needed.

This formula is thick because it incorporates coconut oil and shea butter. Even though it is a rather "greasy" makeup remover, its rich texture will deeply nourish mature, dry skin with essential fatty acids and vitamins.

Anti-Aging Makeup Remover

This formulation calls for a unique blend of oils that will remove heavy makeup, including foundation, eye shadow, and waterproof mascara, while leaving behind very little oily residue. It is also a rich mix that will nourish the skin with essential fatty acids, vitamin E, coenzyme Q10 and other antioxidants that prevent skin aging and wrinkle formation.

INGREDIENTS

1 softgel coenzyme Q10
2 ounces (60 ml) almond oil
1 ounce (30 ml) jojoba oil
1 ounce (30 ml) macadamia oil
1 teaspoon cranberry seed oil
20 drops (1 ml) vitamin E

INSTRUCTIONS

1. Start by puncturing the Q10 softgel with a heated needle and squeezing the contents into a small bowl. Mix with the remaining oils and vitamin E; then transfer to a pump bottle.

2. Wet your face with your fingertips, rub the makeup remover on your face, and then remove your makeup with a cotton disk. Feel free to repeat the process if your face is not satisfactorily clean.

3. Wetting your face with the fingertips will make the oil slip on the skin's surface and spread more easily, requiring a smaller amount of remover and leaving only traces of oily residue.

4. Do not rinse if you want to preserve some of the great anti-aging properties of this formula.

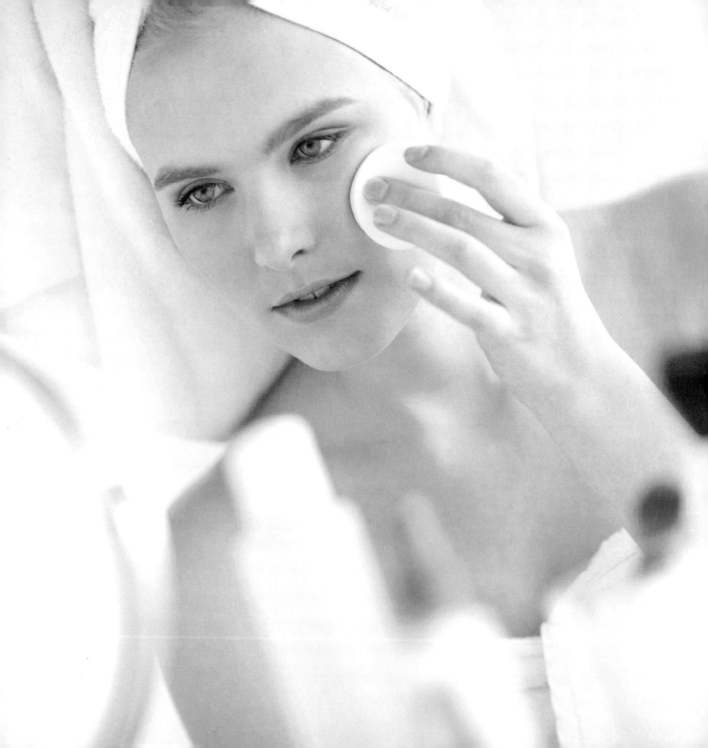

CHAPTER 7

Toners

Toners are thin liquids, with or without alcohol, that are applied to the face and neck, to clear the skin of oily secretions and to remove any makeup traces left behind by a makeup remover. Not all toners are astringent, and not all of them are for oily skin. Some toners are moisturizing, and most of the time, no rinsing is needed.

Making your own toner is very easy and fun. Since toners consist mainly of water and water-soluble ingredients, their minimum complexity makes a nice start for a natural beauty beginner. Always prepare small quantities to make sure your toner stays fresh.

Among the key ingredients are the following:

- Hydrosols, or flower waters. Some hydrosols, such as rose water, bring softening and soothing properties to skin. Others, such as neroli water, might help tame breakouts and provide astringency. Hydrosols are blended with water and other ingredients to make a complete toner.

- Glycerin is a basic ingredient that blends well with most toner formulas. Make sure it is from a vegetable source. Feel free to add it to your favorite toner: 1 tablespoon of glycerin per cup of toner. Because it acts as a skin emollient, glycerin will soften the skin and help preserve its moisture. It also draws moisture to skin from the surrounding air. Its presence in a formulation will give your toner a silkier texture.

- Vitamin E is a natural preservative and an antioxidant. Because toners have very high water content, they need preservation. Adding vitamin

E to your toner will help extend its shelf life while protecting skin from aging by neutralizing free radicals. Add a few drops to the oil phase of your products. Always shake your toner bottle vigorously to disperse the droplets within the liquid before applying it.

- Almond milk can give your toner a smoother texture and add some properties that water alone cannot provide. Almond milk is rich in vitamin E and is easy to mix with aqueous toners. Commercial almond milk is rich in calcium and contains thickeners such as xanthan gum.

Universal Basic Chamomile Toner

Made with one of the most skin-friendly ingredients, this soothing chamomile-based toner is among the easiest to prepare. Use it as is or as a base for more complex formulas. While honey is a time-tested anti-aging ingredient, glycerin will soften the texture of the toner and act as a humectant.

INGREDIENTS

1 cup distilled water

2 tablespoons loose chamomile, or 2 chamomile tea bags

½ teaspoon honey

1 teaspoon glycerin

INSTRUCTIONS

1. Boil 1 cup of distilled water and pour it over the chamomile. Cover and steep for 10 minutes before squeezing and removing tea bags if used, or straining loose tea. Add the honey and glycerin and stir until everything is well blended.

2. Wait for the chamomile infusion to cool before transferring it to a bottle.

3. Apply generously, once or twice a day, to a clean face and neck (and chest, if desired) with a cotton ball. No need to rinse.

Double C Toner

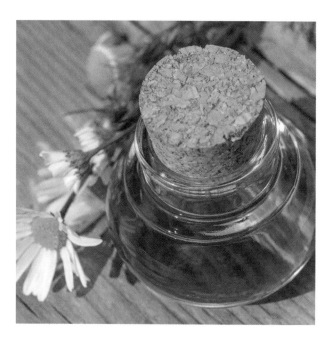

This golden recipe is a chamomile and carrot toner, a very simple and skin-friendly formula that suits all skin types. Because carrots are rich in carotene, which is a precursor of the anti-aging vitamin A, using it on your skin helps boost your skin's vitality while keeping it moisturized in the most gentle fashion.

INGREDIENTS

    1 cup chamomile infusion at room temperature
    ½ cup carrot juice
    1 teaspoon glycerin

INSTRUCTIONS

1. Transfer the chamomile infusion to a bottle. Filter the carrot juice through a strainer and pour it over the chamomile. Add the glycerin and shake vigorously to mix.

2. Shake well before pouring onto a cotton ball to use. Apply to face and neck at bedtime. Wait 5 minutes, then rinse with tepid water.

Vitamins and Minerals Blend

This nourishing formula makes a wonderful summer drink for your skin, especially after you've been sweating in the sun. Watermelon is a known source of vitamins and antioxidants, and Himalayan salt is among the purest salts, unprocessed, and extremely rich in minerals. That is why this "drink" will restore a glow to dull skin. Honey will help moisturize the skin and act as a natural anti-aging agent that will boost the watermelon's efficacy.

INGREDIENTS

2 cups finely diced watermelon

1 cup filtered water

1 tablespoon honey

Pinch of Himalayan sea salt

INSTRUCTIONS

1. Cut the watermelon into pieces, then mash and strain it to get 1 cup of juice.

2. Warm the filtered water in a double boiler; then add the honey, stirring until the honey is completely dissolved. Make sure not to overheat. Add the watermelon juice, sprinkle with salt, stir, and set aside to cool.

3. Transfer to a bottle.

4. Pour onto a cotton ball and apply in the evening to the face and neck to compensate for the skin's loss of moisture after sweating on a hot summer day. Daily use through the summer season is very beneficial for the skin.

Skin-Brightening Toner

Sometimes a toner can do more than just make sure your makeup is gone. A little twist on a basic formula, and—voilà—a bonus benefit unwrapped. Lemons contain high levels of vitamin C, which acts as a skin brightener. Rubbing alcohol (from cologne) is a great solvent for extracting that vitamin C from lemon rind, while helping extend the toner's shelf life and tame skin bacteria. Since sun damage is mostly visible after summer, fall and winter are the best times of the year to reverse that damage and rejuvenate the skin. Adding water will bring down the final alcohol level of this toner, and a touch of glycerin will help counteract its drying effect.

INGREDIENTS

1 lemon rind
½ cup mild cologne (such as baby cologne)
1 cup water
1 teaspoon glycerin

Note: You can substitute grapefruit or orange peel for the lemon rind.

INSTRUCTIONS

1. Put the lemon rind in a glass jar, pour the cologne over it, close the jar, and leave for 3–5 days in a cool place and away from sunlight, shaking occasionally.

2. Filter the cologne through a strainer, add 1 cup of water, then the glycerin, shake well, and transfer to a bottle.

3. Apply to clean skin at bedtime. Wait for 5 minutes before rinsing with water.

4. Daily use of sunscreen is essential to prevent skin photosensitivity.

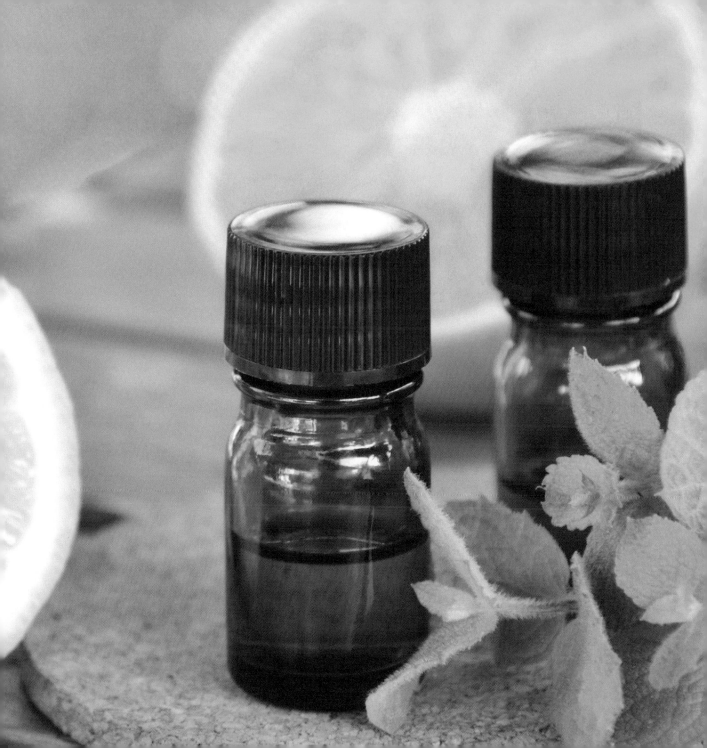

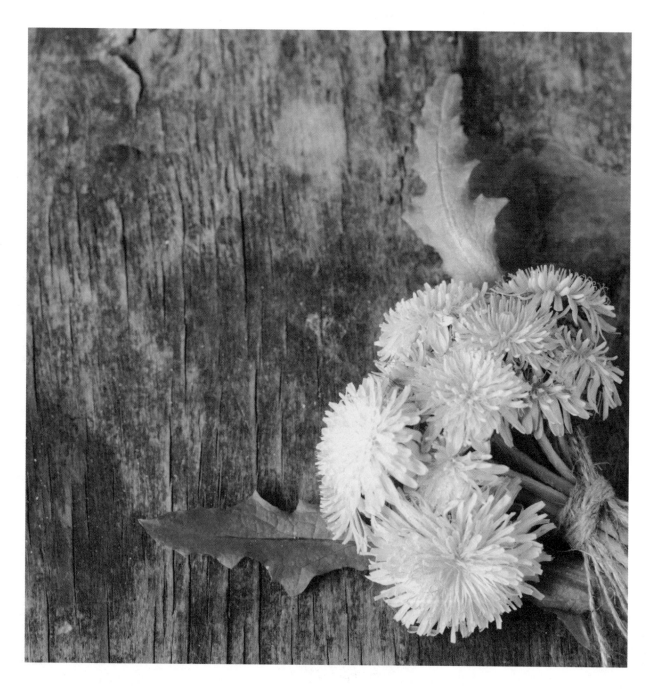

Herbal Toner

Dandelion is a highly praised herb that offers uncountable benefits. It is among the top-ranked herbs in Chinese herbal medicine. It is extremely rich in vitamin A, as well as vitamins B and C and many minerals, such as iron, phosphorus, magnesium, calcium, zinc, and copper. As a topical ingredient, it will improve skin vitality and tonus for a more youthful appearance. The addition of rose water, an uplifting, skin-friendly ingredient, makes this a gently soothing toner that you can enjoy year round.

INGREDIENTS

2 heaping tablespoons chopped dandelion greens

1 cup hot water

1 ounce (30 ml) rose water

1 teaspoon glycerin

INSTRUCTIONS

1. Prepare an infusion of the chopped dandelion and hot water. Strain out the leaves, making sure to squeeze out excess liquid, and set aside to cool.

2. Add the rose water and glycerin. Stir well and transfer to a bottle.

3. Use a cotton ball to apply twice a day to a clean face and neck.

Flowery Toner

This wonderfully scented toner will add a pleasing component to your morning routine. Simple, skin friendly, with an uplifting fragrance, it clarifies, cleans, and moisturizes the skin. The addition of the antioxidant, anti-aging vitamin E increases the benefits conferred by this toner.

INGREDIENTS

2 tablespoons roughly chopped rose petals

2 tablespoons geranium petals (or lavender, according to availability)

1 cup water

1 teaspoon glycerin

1 teaspoon baby cologne

20 drops (1 ml) vitamin E

INSTRUCTIONS

1. In a glass bowl, blend the flower petals. Boil the water and pour it over the petals. Cover the bowl, wrap it with a towel to keep the heat in, and set it aside.

2. Try to rotate the bowl clockwise, then counter-clockwise, every 30 minutes to shake things a bit and encourage fragrance transfer.

3. After about 3 hours of contact time, strain the petals out of the liquid, making sure to squeeze out excess liquid trapped within the petals. Then add remaining ingredients.

4. Shake to mix and transfer to a bottle.

5. Shake again prior to using, and apply with a cotton ball. Use in the morning for softer and delicately scented skin.

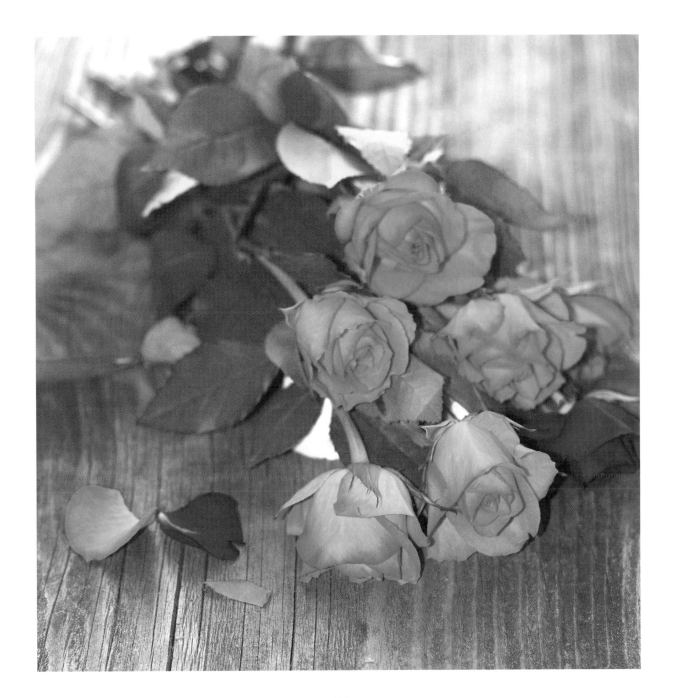

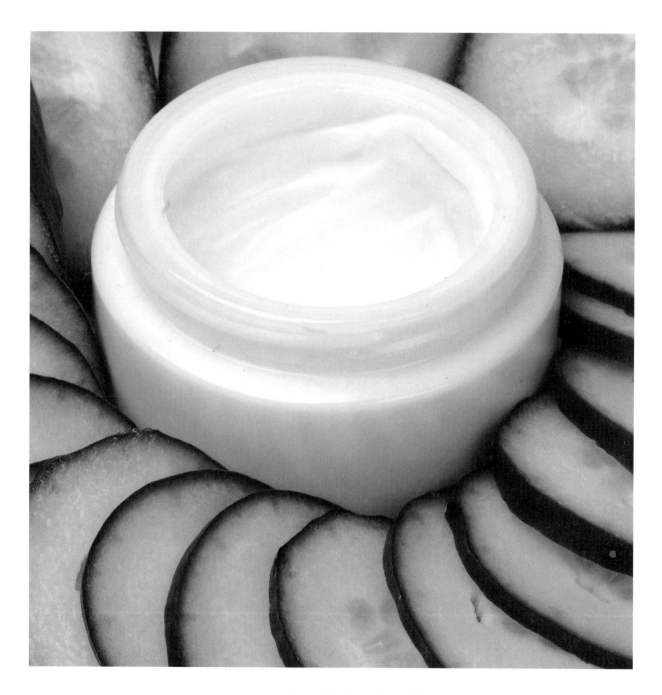

Creamy Toner

Dry skin usually lacks moisture, and since an oily film on the skin surface locks moisture underneath it, thick, oil-rich ingredients are suitable for drier skin.

Heavy cream provides a "shot" of lipids for dry skin. With other moisturizing ingredients, such as glycerin, cucumber juice, and honey, this toner is a perfect balance for weather-beaten skin. Buying organic, when it's available, helps you avoid pesticides, antibiotics, and hormones in your ingredients.

INGREDIENTS

1 English cucumber

½ cup heavy cream

1 ounce (30 ml) rose water

1 teaspoon vegetable glycerin

1 teaspoon honey

Note: Aloe vera juice or gel can be substituted for the cucumber juice, 1 tablespoon cologne for the 2 tablespoons rose water, and almond milk for the cream (for a nongreasy formulation).

INSTRUCTIONS

1. Make cucumber juice by putting 1 English cucumber through a juicer. Filter the cucumber juice, and then mix with the heavy cream. Warm the rose water in a double boiler; then add the honey and stir to dissolve. Add the glycerin to the rose water and honey and mix again. Pour over the cucumber juice and cream mixture. Then transfer to a bottle.

2. Shake vigorously to combine all ingredients. Store in the refrigerator for up to a week or to the cream's expiration date, whichever is shorter.

3. Shake again before applying to the face and neck with a cotton ball before bedtime.

Almond Milk and Olive Oil Toner

Heavier oils, such as olive or avocado, are a great choice for dry skin. Olive oil is rich in unsaturated fatty acids, and its consistency provides durable protection against aggressive weather and moisture loss. Even though it is optional, the addition of evening primrose oil is a big bonus, because it confers anti-aging properties to this formula.

INGREDIENTS

½ cup almond milk

½ cup distilled water

1 ounce (30 ml) olive oil

1 ounce (30 ml) rose water

20 drops (1 ml) evening primrose oil (optional)

10 drops (0.5 ml) vitamin E

INSTRUCTIONS

1. Combine all ingredients in a bottle. Shake vigorously to mix, and store in the refrigerator for up to a week.

2. Separation is to be expected. Always shake the bottle vigorously before applying this toner, in the evening, to the face and neck with a cotton ball or disk.

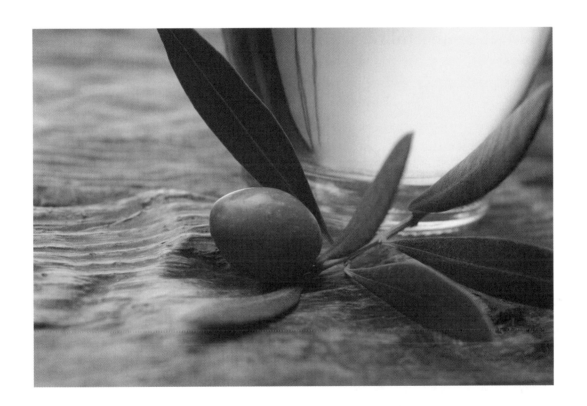

Almond Rose Toner

This toner is very easy to make and produces wonderful results.

It moisturizes and softens skin without leaving an oily residue. That is mainly because of the composition of jojoba oil, which is very close to that of skin oils. That is why jojoba is a big-time favorite in skin care products.

INGREDIENTS

½ cup almond milk

½ cup rose water

1 tablespoon jojoba oil

1 teaspoon glycerin

10 drops (0.5 ml) vitamin E

INSTRUCTIONS

1. Combine all the ingredients in a bottle. Shake vigorously to blend well.

2. You can store this toner in the refrigerator for up to a week.

3. Always shake prior to application to disperse the oil droplets. Soak a cotton ball with this toner and wipe the face and neck daily.

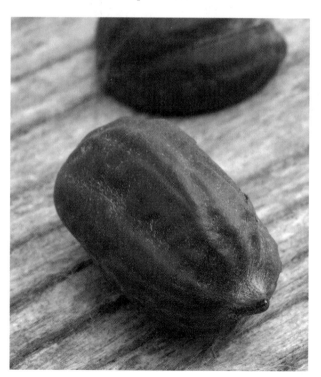

Kaolin Astringent Toner

Many of the ingredients in this formula, such as tea tree oil and witch hazel, contribute to its astringent effect. Kaolin, also called china clay, will give body to your toner while drawing oils and toxins away from the skin surface. Tea tree oil is also an antiseptic, which helps limit bacterial proliferation. Wheat germ is extremely nourishing and provides anti-aging benefits; it is added as a powder to keep the formula oil free. This wholesome formula is excellent for oily skin that needs cleaning, astringency, and nourishment.

INGREDIENTS

1 teaspoon white kaolin

1 teaspoon wheat germ powder

½ cup witch hazel water

10 drops (0.5 ml) tea tree essential oil

INSTRUCTIONS

1. Start by mixing the dry ingredients, kaolin and wheat germ, then gradually add that mixture to the witch hazel, stirring thoroughly to make sure your preparation is well blended. Finally, add the tea tree oil; then mix and transfer to a bottle.

2. Remember to always shake the bottle prior to using. Apply a quarter-size amount to a wet face and neck, and wait 3–5 minutes before rinsing it off with tepid water. Do not rub, because excessive rubbing might stimulate the sebaceous glands and lead to more oily secretions.

3. This formula can be used every morning during breakouts.

Cucumber Toner

Cucumber is a very lightweight moisturizer, suitable and refreshing for sensitive skin. Rely on its juice to clean skin without clogging pores. The slight amount of rubbing alcohol from cologne helps clear skin and tame bacteria. Tea tree oil is also antiseptic and offers a complementary astringent effect.

INGREDIENTS

½ English cucumber

1 tablespoon cologne

½ cup water

1 teaspoon glycerin

10 drops (0.5 ml) tea tree oil

INSTRUCTIONS

1. Peel and chop fresh cucumber, then puree with a stick blender. Add cologne to the cucumber puree, then dilute with ½ cup water and let stand for 2 hours.

2. Filter through a strainer; then add the glycerin and tea tree oil and transfer to a bottle.

3. Shake well before using. Soak a cotton ball and apply to the face and décolletage in the morning, for a noticeably clearer skin.

Evening Tea Toner

This formula is concocted with very basic ingredients that provide remarkable benefits. Black tea contains tannins and acts as an astringent, which makes it a wonderful choice for oily skin, reducing sebum production and tightening pores. Lemon juice helps improve the appearance of blemishes, and the little amount of rubbing alcohol from cologne reduces bacterial proliferation and helps clear skin.

INGREDIENTS

½ cup hot water

1 tea bag or 1 tablespoon loose black tea

1 teaspoon lemon juice

1 tablespoon baby cologne

INSTRUCTIONS

1. Pour the hot water over the tea. Cover and leave for 30 minutes.

2. Squeeze excess liquid from the tea bag before removing it, or strain loose tea; add lemon juice and allow further cooling.

3. Add cologne when mixture is completely cooled, right before transferring it to a bottle, to avoid alcohol evaporation.

4. Soak a cotton ball and roll it over the face and neck every evening.

5. Daily use of sunscreen is strongly advised, as this recipe can increase photosensitivity.

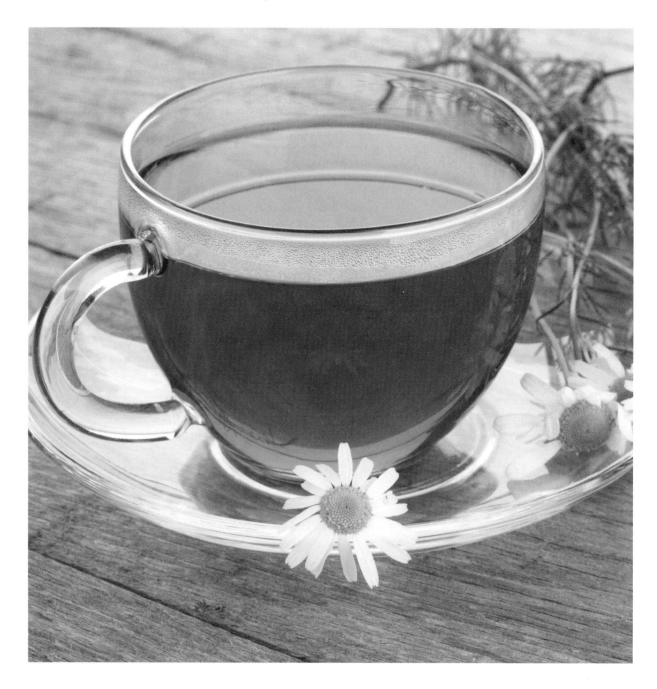

Astringent Toner

This formula combines the astringent properties of both black tea and witch hazel for maximum efficacy in reducing sebum production in acne-prone skin. It also calls for the antiseptic powers of rubbing alcohol. This is an acidic formulation that will help clear skin and improve the appearance of blemishes.

INGREDIENTS

½ cup black tea

½ cup witch hazel water

1 tablespoon apple cider vinegar

1 tablespoon baby cologne

INSTRUCTIONS

1. Prepare a regular cup of black tea. Enjoy half and save ½ cup to prepare this toner. Allow it to cool to room temperature. When it has reached room temperature, add all remaining ingredients, stir, and transfer to a bottle.

2. Soak a cotton ball with this toner and apply to oily facial zones by dabbing once a day—without excessive rubbing to prevent overstimulation of sebaceous glands and a rebound effect. Rinse thoroughly and remember daily application of sunscreen.

Double C Toner for Acne-Prone Skin

This toner is named for its two key ingredients: vitamin C and cider. The acidic nature of apple cider allows skin to get rid of surface dead cells, while the vitamin C in lemon juice is a skin brightener that also acts as a powerful antioxidant; it can reverse sun damage and reduce wrinkles, for a more youthful look. Combined with the astringency of neroli and witch hazel in this formula, they will reduce oily secretions and help achieve a glowing and clearer skin.

INGREDIENTS

1 teaspoon honey

½ cup water

2 ounces (60 ml) neroli hydrosol

2 ounces (60 ml) witch hazel water

1 tablespoon apple cider

1 tablespoon lemon juice

1 teaspoon glycerin

5 drops grapefruit essential oil (optional)

INSTRUCTIONS

1. Start by dissolving the honey in ½ cup water. Add the remaining ingredients one at a time, mixing continuously. Then transfer to a bottle.

2. Shake well before each use. Using a cotton ball, apply to the face and neck in the evening. Rinse in the morning and wear sunscreen daily.

Tea Tree Oil Toner

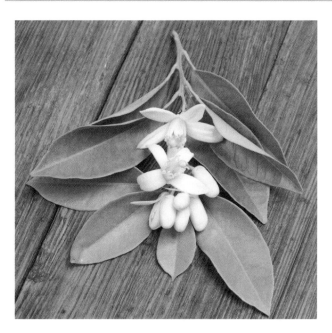

INGREDIENTS

2 ounces (60 ml) aloe vera juice

1 teaspoon royal jelly

2 ounces (60 ml) orange blossom water

1 teaspoon apple cider

1 teaspoon vegetable glycerin

10 drops (0.5 ml) tea tree essential oil

1 teaspoon hazelnut oil

INSTRUCTIONS

1. Start by pouring the aloe vera juice over the royal jelly, whisking to dissolve the jelly. Add the orange blossom water, making sure all the jelly is dissolved. Add the apple cider and glycerin, and whisk again.

2. In a separate bowl, add the tea tree oil to the hazelnut oil, mix, and then add to the first mixture, whisking continuously until well blended. Transfer to a bottle and shake very well to disperse the essential oil.

3. Always shake the bottle vigorously prior to application to disperse the oils. Apply with a cotton ball to reduce blemishes on the face, chest, and upper back, preferably at bedtime. Allow at least 5 minutes contact time before rinsing.

4. Daily use of sunscreen is always recommended.

This complete formula is specifically suitable for acne-prone skin.

It incorporates multiple ingredients that work together for maximum sebum control (tea tree oil, neroli water, and hazelnut oil) while providing moisture (glycerin and aloe vera) and wholesome nutrients (royal jelly). This is a wonderfully scented toner whose uplifting bright fragrance you can enjoy while taming breakouts.

Sage Infusion Toner

Since sage has anti-inflammatory properties very similar to those of aspirin, or salicylates, a sage infusion can be extremely helpful in soothing skin redness. Make sure, however, that you seek a medical opinion for your skin condition prior to applying this toner.

INGREDIENTS

1 cup hot distilled water

1 tablespoon fresh or dried sage

1 teaspoon glycerin

INSTRUCTIONS

1. Pour the water over the sage. Cover for 30 minutes. Then strain out the leaves and set the liquid aside to cool.

2. Add the glycerin, whisk to blend, and transfer to a spray bottle.

3. Apply gently using a cotton ball, or spray directly on irritated skin. Do not rub.

4. The cool temperature will help reduce dilation of blood vessels and decrease redness. Repeat 2–3 times daily to soothe skin.

5. Store the bottle in the refrigerator for up to a week.

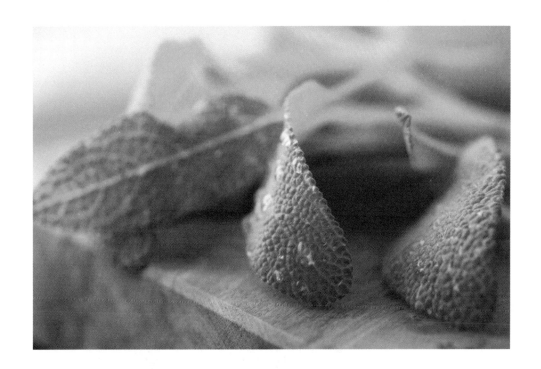

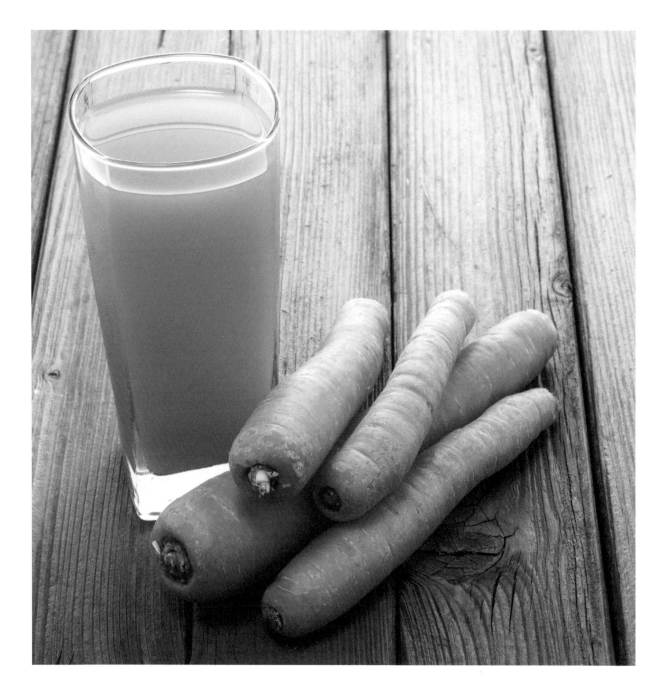

Calming Toner for Irritated Skin

This formula relies on the anti-inflammatory properties of sage and rosemary, which will help soothe inflamed skin. While fresh herbs are always best, dried will also work. Carrot juice is added to provide carotenoids, which will give a healthier look to tired skin. Rose water is also a universal soother, very gentle on all skin types. Together those ingredients will work in harmony to help you achieve a soothed and revived skin.

INGREDIENTS

1 teaspoon sage

1 teaspoon rosemary

3 ounces (100 ml) distilled water

1 tablespoon carrot juice

2 ounces (60 ml) rose water

INSTRUCTIONS

1. Mix sage and rosemary in a mug or glass beaker. Pour 3 ounces freshly boiled water over them and cover. After 10 minutes, strain out the herbs and set the liquid aside to cool.

2. Meanwhile, pour the carrot juice into a spray bottle. Pour the herbal tea over the carrot juice and finish by adding the rose water. Shake the bottle vigorously to mix well.

3. Spray lightly onto the face and neck 2–3 times daily.

4. No need for rinsing or drying with a towel; rubbing is also not recommended, because it might cause further irritation.

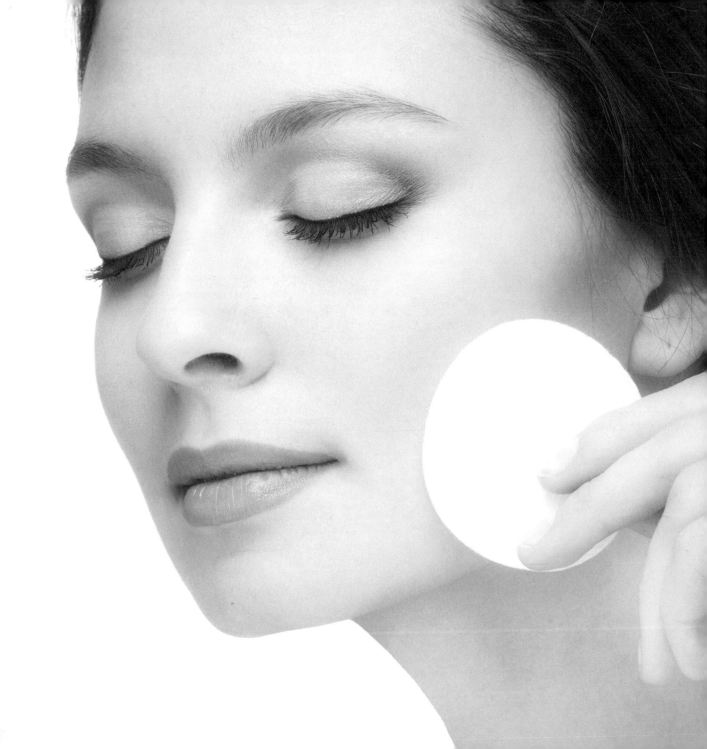

CHAPTER 8

Evening Oils and Serums

Night is the time when the body recovers from the challenges of the day. While day creams provide moisture and shield skin from sun damage, night creams and oils target skin nutrition and wrinkle prevention. If you want to nurture your skin at night, give it more nutrients and well-chosen evening oils for fabulous results.

3-in-1 Lazy Blend

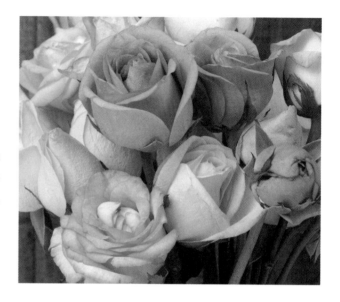

What could be better than a makeup remover that is also a toner and an anti-aging night oil all in one bottle? This formula softens the skin and nourishes it. While the composition of jojoba oil is very close to that of the skin's own lipids and it doesn't clog pores, wheat germ oil is rich in vitamins and minerals that prevent aging. Chamomile tea and rose water are extremely skin friendly and help, alongside glycerin, balance moisture levels. Keep this oil-water mix handy, especially when you have little time and energy left at the end of the day.

INGREDIENTS

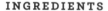

2 ounces (60 ml) rose water

1 tablespoon almond oil

1 tablespoon jojoba oil

1 tablespoon wheat germ

1 ounce (30 ml) chamomile tea (at room temperature)

1 teaspoon glycerin

5 drops vitamin E oil

Note: You can substitute witch hazel for rose water in case of oily skin.

INSTRUCTIONS

1. Mix the above ingredients, adding one at a time. Shake well, and then transfer to a spray bottle.

2. Shake vigorously to disperse oil droplets before spraying onto a cotton disc or ball. Wipe the face and neck, repeating if necessary to remove makeup completely.

3. You do not need to rinse or follow with a toner or night oil, because this formula does it all.

4. Store the bottle in a cool place away from sunlight and heat.

Precious Night Oil

Rosehip oil is a great anti-aging oil, rich in GLA, LA, and other essential fatty acids, as well as vitamin A and E. Together with essential oils, which impart a pleasant scent, those ingredients provide this simple formula with most of what skin needs to be adequately nurtured. Prepare this formula to help mature skin fight wrinkles.

INGREDIENTS

1 tablespoon rosehip oil

1 tablespoon sunflower oil

5 drops gardenia essential oil (or other)

10 drops (0.5 ml) vitamin E oil

INSTRUCTIONS

1. Mix all the above ingredients and transfer to an amber bottle with a dropper.

2. After removing all makeup traces, and while skin is still moist from cleansing, spread 2–3 drops all over your face and neck every night. Store away from heat and direct sunlight.

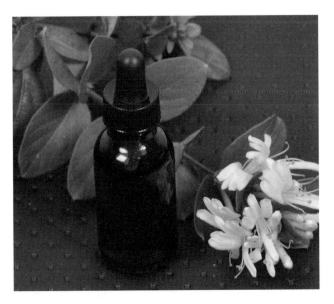

Night Magic Potion

This "potion" indeed works like magic. It fights wrinkles, nourishes skin, and leaves a velvety touch in the morning. While avocado oil is rich in vitamin E and essential fatty acids, evening primrose oil is a powerful anti-aging ingredient that fights wrinkles. Their efficacy is made complete with the addition of pomegranate seed oil, which provides a surge of antioxidants that protect from sun damage and promote youthful-looking skin. Grapefruit or tangerine essential oil transforms the application of this potion into a pleasurable moment. The essential oils may be photosensitizing, however, so daily use of sunblock is strongly recommended.

INGREDIENTS

1 tablespoon avocado oil

1 tablespoon evening primrose oil

1 tablespoon pomegranate seed oil

1 tablespoon almond oil

1 tablespoon sunflower oil

10 drops (0.5 ml) essential oil of your choice (grapefruit, tangerine, or other)

INSTRUCTIONS

1. Mix the above ingredients in their listed order and transfer to a glass bottle with a dropper.

2. Make sure your face is clean, with no makeup residue, and still moist after cleansing or washing. Rub a few drops of this potion between your palms and pat your face and neck. Do not rinse.

3. Use every evening at bedtime. Store the bottle away from heat and light.

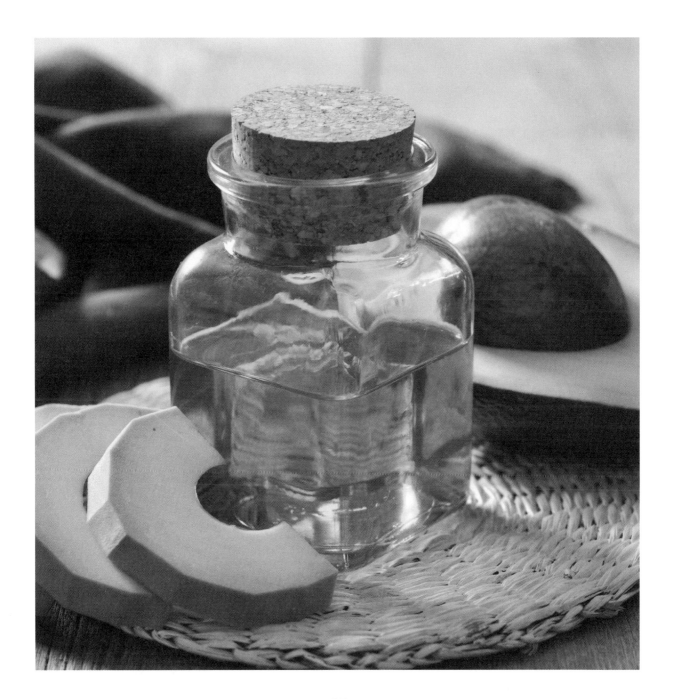

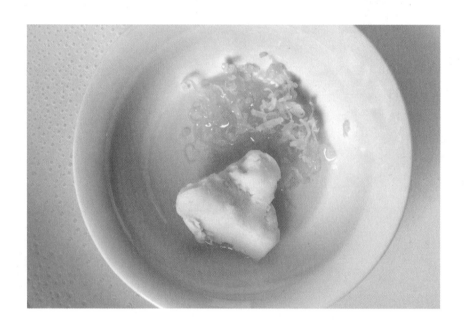

Anti-Aging Rosehip Balm

This powerful formula combines the highly prized anti-aging effects of rosehip oil with the moisture-locking properties of beeswax. Shea butter is also a key player in this formula, since it is a powerful skin-softening agent. Not intended for daily routine, this balm is especially recommended for dry and mature skin, when an SOS rescue is needed, such as to counteract cold weather aggression on skin.

INGREDIENTS

1 tablespoon grated unrefined, unbleached beeswax

1 ounce (30 ml) shea butter

2 ounces (60 ml) almond oil

20 drops (1 ml) vitamin E

1 tablespoon rosehip oil

10 drops (0.5 ml) rose or geranium essential oil

INSTRUCTIONS

1. Melt the beeswax and shea butter in a double boiler. Then add the almond oil and vitamin E. Turn off the heat and then add the rosehip oil. Do not overheat the rosehip oil to preserve its properties. Add the essential oil last.

2. Stir continuously until the mixture cools to room temperature. Transfer to a glass jar or a tin box and leave in a cool place to solidify. Cover with a lid when the balm is completely cool.

3. Apply with the fingertips to a well-cleansed face and neck every evening. Dab around the eye area without pulling the skin. You do not need to rinse. Enjoy a rejuvenated, silky soft skin in the morning.

4. Please note that this formula is not recommended for prolonged use because beeswax is considered comedogenic and can clog pores.

Sensitive Skin Anti-Aging Serum

This unscented oily serum is especially formulated for intolerant skin; it's suitable for most skin types, however, and is a powerful moisturizer, packed with antioxidants. Sesame oil is a skin-friendly oil, well-tolerated by most skin types, even the most sensitive ones; it contains sesamol, which has antioxidant properties, as well as unsaturated essential fatty acids and many minerals such as magnesium, calcium, and iron. Grape seed oil is also a strong source of antioxidants and is a dry oil that absorbs quickly. This formula is kept simple by calling for ingredients that can be found in most grocery stores.

INGREDIENTS

1 tablespoon sesame oil

1 tablespoon grape seed oil

1 tablespoon sunflower oil

5 drops vitamin E oil

INSTRUCTIONS

1. Pour the oils into a glass bottle with a dropper, finishing with the vitamin E drops.

2. Close tightly and shake to blend the oils.

3. In the evening, after cleansing, and while the face is still moist, apply 2–3 drops to your hands, rub them together, and massage this serum onto your face and neck.

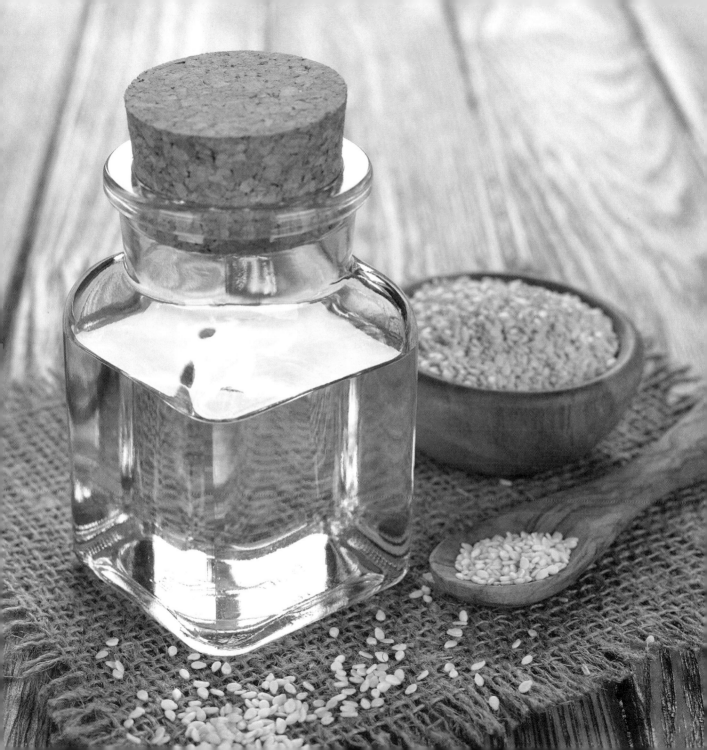

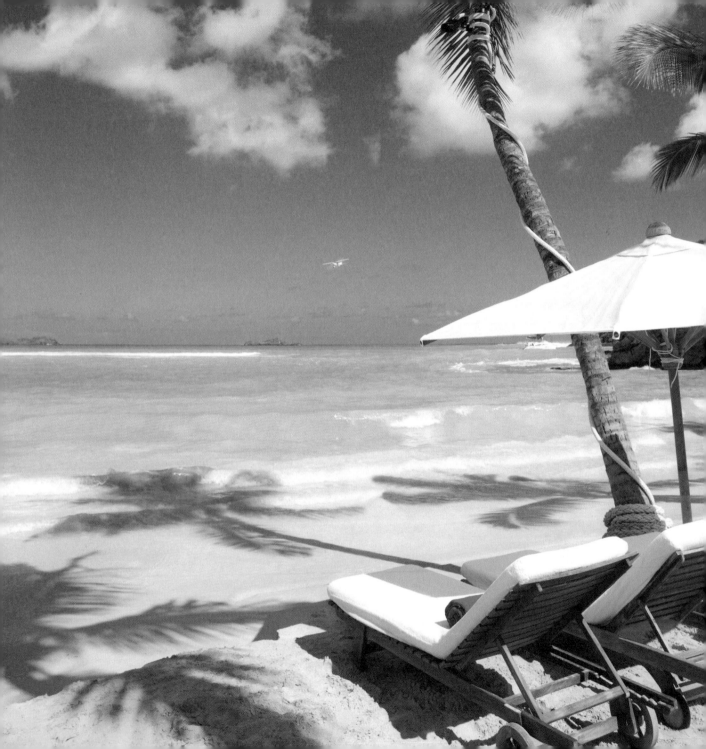

CHAPTER 9

Facial Creams and Sunscreen

You should be very proud of yourself when you feel ready to make your first cream. The biggest challenge in making creams is achieving a nice texture and lasting stability. Sometimes creams can be runny. They can also separate or turn out gritty. This very delicate process is perfectly doable if you start with a good base formula and follow it with accuracy.

Every cream has a base. Additives can vary, but the heart of the cream remains the same: an oil phase, an aqueous phase, and something that binds the two: an emulsifier. Generally speaking, if the oil phase is waxy or buttery (solid at room temperature), then your cream will thicken as it cools. But if you start with liquids, the final texture will remain liquid unless you use a thickener.

It is very convenient to use a thickening emulsifier that gives body and texture to the formulation, as well. Also, the adequate use of a thickener will improve stability and reduce the risk of separation.

Once you have mastered the base of your cream, substituting oils or adding botanical extracts will become easier. You will then be able to create a customized cream that targets your own skin needs.

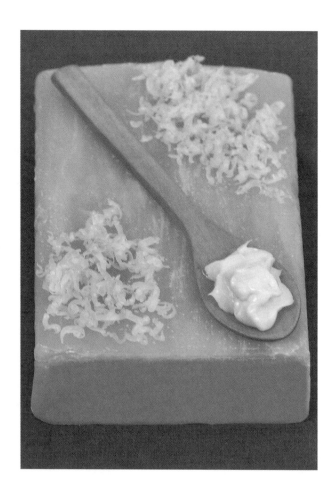

Beeswax Facial Cream

Beeswax is a natural emulsifier and a thickener. As your preparation cools, beeswax will solidify, and your cream will thicken. At the same time, beeswax locks in moisture by acting as a water barrier. On the other hand, it confers a greasy finish to the cream, which is why it is more suitable for dry skin. If you find that your cream's texture is cosmetically unappealing, a lesser amount of beeswax usually solves the issue.

INGREDIENTS

- 1 ounce (30 ml) unbleached, unrefined beeswax, grated
- 2 ounces (60 ml) almond oil
- 20 drops (1 ml) vitamin E oil
- 1 ounce (30 ml) water or hydrosol, such as rose water
- 20 drops (1 ml) botanical extract such as watermelon
- 4 drops rosemary oil extract (as a preservative)
- 20 drops (1 ml) essential oils of your choice

INSTRUCTIONS

1. Melt the wax in a double boiler. Without taking the wax off the heat, add the oily ingredients (almond oil and vitamin E) to the melted beeswax, one at a time, whisking continuously.

2. In a separate double boiler, heat the hydrosol until it reaches 175° F. Monitor the temperature using a candy thermometer. Wait until both phases have reached that temperature; then turn off the heat and slowly pour the water phase over the wax in a very thin stream, whisking vigorously. You can use a stick blender for better results.

3. Keep mixing while the preparation starts to cool and as you add the remaining ingredients one at a time. Transfer to a sanitized glass jar, and set aside to cool completely to room temperature. Put a lid on the jar when your cream is no longer warm.

4. Apply as a night cream during winter, alternating with a lighter cream (such as the Basic Cream, page 150) to allow your skin to breathe.

Basic Cream

This lighter cream that does not contain beeswax makes a good basic formula for a moisturizer.

As long as you respect the proportions, you can play with ingredients to create a cream that suits your own skin needs. You can choose a single herbal extract or a blend of two or more to gain additional skin benefits—for example, use alfalfa extract for its anti-aging properties with licorice extract for its whitening effect.

The texture of the cream can also be adjusted. Use only oils for a lighter texture, or a blend of oils and butters for a thicker cream. The oils and extracts you choose will impart their own properties to the finished cream.

Making creams may require many attempts before you can predict how your ingredients will blend and bond together. If your cream expels water, you need to use less hydrosol. If it is too hard, you need less butter and more oil. If your cream is closer to a lotion than a cream, you need less water and more thickener. Prepare small batches, until you are able to master this art.

INGREDIENTS

1 ounce (30 ml) vegetable oil or shea butter

2 teaspoons vegetable-derived emulsifier, such as lecithin or glyceryl stearate

10 drops (0.5 ml) vitamin E oil

2 ounces (60 ml) water or hydrosol, such as rose water

20 drops (1 ml) botanical extract, such as pomegranate seed extract

3 drops rosemary oil extract (ROE) or grape seed extract (GSE)

10 drops (0.5 ml) essential oils

NOTE

When using oils only, a good thickener is essential. Xanthan gum at 0.3 percent can transform the water phase into a gel, which is more stable in an emulsion than water. Sprinkle gum on your water phase before adding the oils. Start with a pinch and observe the result upon whisking. Usually, ¼ teaspoon xanthan gum is sufficient to thicken the mixture. A little trick that might help is to use aloe vera gel instead of a liquid hydrosol for easier thickening.

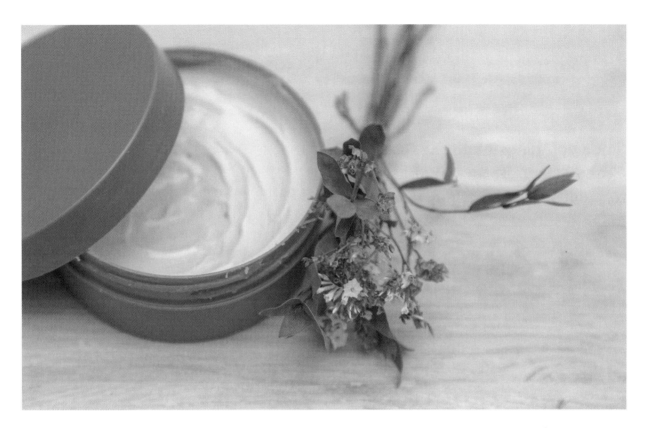

INSTRUCTIONS

1. Melt the butter or heat the vegetable oil in a double boiler over low heat. Mix in the vegetable-derived emulsifier and vitamin E, stirring continuously.

2. Heat the water phase, the hydrosol, in another double boiler. If your botanical extract is stable at high temperature, you can incorporate it into your water phase. Otherwise, leave it aside for later.

3. Monitor the temperature using a candy thermometer. When both phases reach 170°F turn off the heat and pour the oil phase, in a thin stream, over the water phase, whisking vigorously, or use a stick blender, avoiding splashes.

4. The mixture should blend into a whitish creamy texture. Keep whipping until the mixture reaches 100°F.

5. Add the extracts and the essential oils and whisk until thoroughly blended. Transfer to a jar and allow to cool to room temperature. Put a lid on the jar when the mixture is no longer warm.

Mineral Sunblock

Once you have made the Basic Cream, (Page 150) you are ready to push things a little further and make a sunscreen. It is also possible to make sunscreen from ready-made natural cream.

Commercial sunscreens are formulated with either chemical filters or mineral filters. Mineral

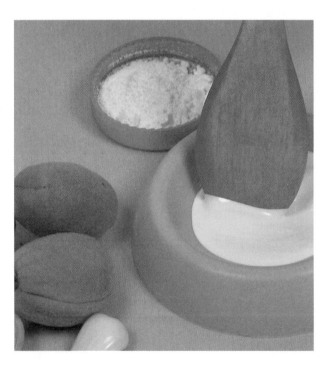

filters, such as zinc oxide and titanium dioxide, are much more stable than chemical filters and do not pose similar health risks. Zinc oxide and titanium dioxide have an indefinite shelf life, which means that they are extremely stable and can tolerate UV light, heat, and moisture without disintegration.

There are different kinds of zinc oxide and titanium dioxide. Micronized particles (in the micron size range) are safer than nano particles (in the nano size range), which have generated health concerns because of their increased potential for absorption through the skin.

The amount of zinc oxide and titanium dioxide in a cream affects the SPF, or sun protection factor. SPF 15 means that it takes fifteen times more UV radiation to burn your skin when it's covered with sunscreen of that strength than it takes when your skin is unprotected. SPF is not a percentage; it is a factor, a number of folds. The average SPF protection is around 15, a sunblock with SPF 30 or more usually provides stronger protection.

Roughly, 10 percent zinc oxide will yield an SPF close to 15, while a 20.5 percent concentration should produce a sunscreen in the SPF 30 range. The SPF varies with the kind of zinc oxide used and the thickness of the formula, as well as the amount spread on the skin. Also, the presence of lumps of zinc oxide in the cream might affect its overall distribution and SPF; it is very important to obtain a well-blended cream and to spread generous amounts on sun-exposed areas.

This formula aims at SPF 30.

INGREDIENTS

21 grams zinc oxide powder

1 tablespoon (15 ml) almond oil

65 grams Basic Cream (sufficient for 100 grams total)

Note: This formula requires a digital scale.

INSTRUCTIONS

1. Sift the zinc oxide into a small mixing bowl. Make sure you do not inhale any of the powder.

2. Add the almond oil, and triturate with a pestle or spoon until a very smooth, lump-free, white paste is obtained.

3. You need just enough Basic Cream to bring the paste weight to an exact 100 grams. Weigh 65 grams and fold gradually, in tiny amounts, into the mixing bowl. Use the same pestle to triturate. Make sure you have no lumps in your sunscreen before you transfer it to a glass container with a lid.

4. Apply generously on your face and neck daily. Do not spread it too thin, as that might compromise the SPF. You can wear mineral makeup on top of the sunscreen to minimize its whitish appearance.

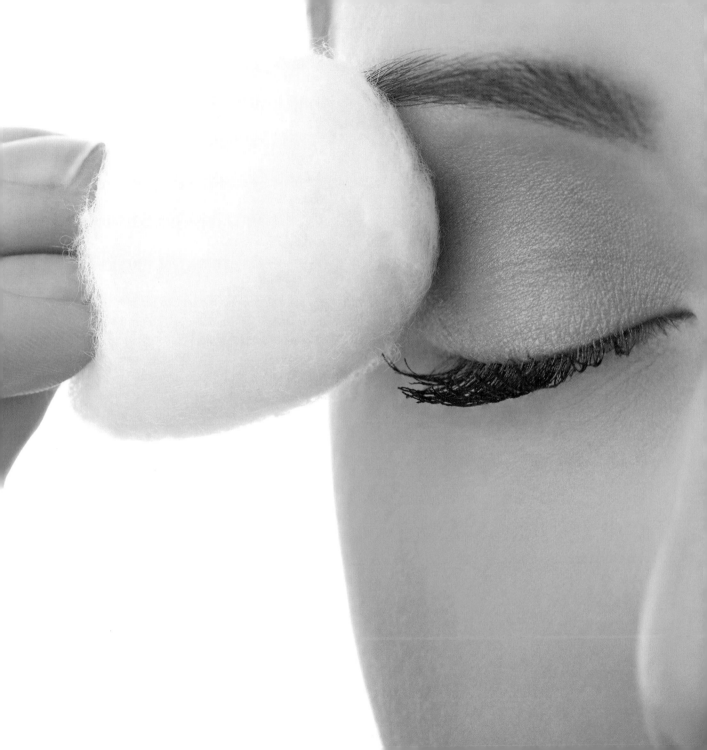

CHAPTER 10

Eye Care

The area surrounding the eyes is very sensitive and requires special care. It is imperative to be diligent regarding makeup removal, wrinkle prevention, dark circles, and puffy eyelids.

Proper hygiene and cleanliness are crucial when preparing eye products. Sanitize your utensils, bottles, droppers, and jars (in the dishwasher on the high-heat cycle), then rinse them with rubbing alcohol and allow it to evaporate. Always clean your work area with rubbing alcohol.

Prepare small amounts, use the products within the indicated time range when given, and discard any remainder after that time, as it may no longer be safe to apply around the eye area.

Eye Makeup Remover

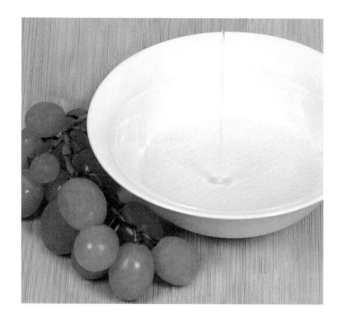

This formula is much more than a simple makeup remover. This blend of oils rich in antioxidants and vitamin E will remove stubborn makeup while nourishing the delicate skin around the eyes and preventing wrinkles. Castor oil, which can be used alone with a Q-tip to remove eyeliner, will promote healthier and longer eyelashes. It has, however, a thick texture, and blending it with dry oils will soften the final consistency. Wheat germ oil is rich in antioxidants and helps prevent wrinkles.

Because this product will be in close contact with the eyes, make sure you maintain a high hygiene level while working, to prevent contamination with germs. This formulation is kept fragrance-free to minimize irritation.

INGREDIENTS

1 tablespoon castor oil

1 tablespoon wheat germ oil

1 tablespoon grape seed oil

10 drops (0.5 ml) vitamin E.

Note: Although wheat germ oil is preferred, you can substitute almond oil if it's unavailable.

INSTRUCTIONS

1. Whisk the top three oils together; then add the vitamin E and transfer the mixture to a sanitized amber bottle with a dropper. Put the top on tightly and shake well.

2. To use, pour a few drops on a cotton ball and wipe off your makeup. Repeat if necessary. Wipe your eyelids gently without pulling the skin.

3. Follow with a toner or a rinse if you do not like the after-feel.

Puffy Eyelids Tea Bags

This title says it all. Black tea is astringent and contains tannins, which help reduce eyelid puffiness.

INGREDIENTS

2 black tea bags

1 cup hot water

1 tablespoon cucumber juice, refrigerated

INSTRUCTIONS

1. Drop the black tea bags into the hot water. Remove after five minutes and let the excess water drain in a bowl while you wait for the bags to cool enough to become comfortable to the touch.

2. Close your eyes and place a tea bag on each eyelid. Relax for 10–15 minutes, flipping the tea bags over every few minutes. Repeat if desired.

3. Finish by gently wiping the eyelids with the cool cucumber juice. Then follow with your usual eye cream.

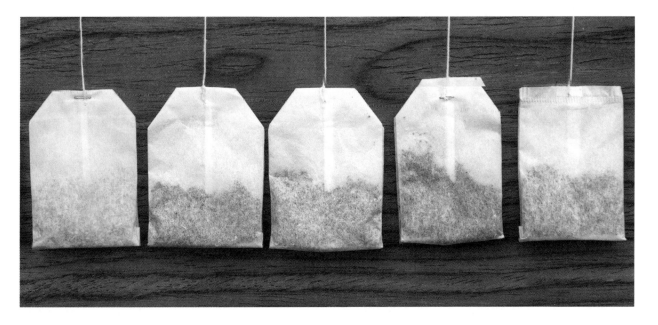

Blue Cornflower Water

This beautiful blue flower (known as bleuet in French) has long been used to make a natural mild astringent and eye antiseptic water. Steam distillation is generally used to make this simple alcohol-free, natural eye toner, but a homemade cornflower infusion will also bring you wonderful results.

INGREDIENTS

1 cup distilled water

1 heaping tablespoon roughly chopped blue cornflower

INSTRUCTIONS

1. Boil the water and pour it over the chopped cornflower into a small bowl. Cover the bowl and wait for 15 minutes, then strain twice through a sanitized cotton cloth or cheesecloth.

2. Transfer the infusion to a sanitized bottle, and close with a lid when it has reached room temperature.

3. To use, pour onto a cotton ball and gently wipe the eyelids, daily after eye makeup removal.

4. Keep refrigerated for up to a week and do not purposely introduce into the eye.

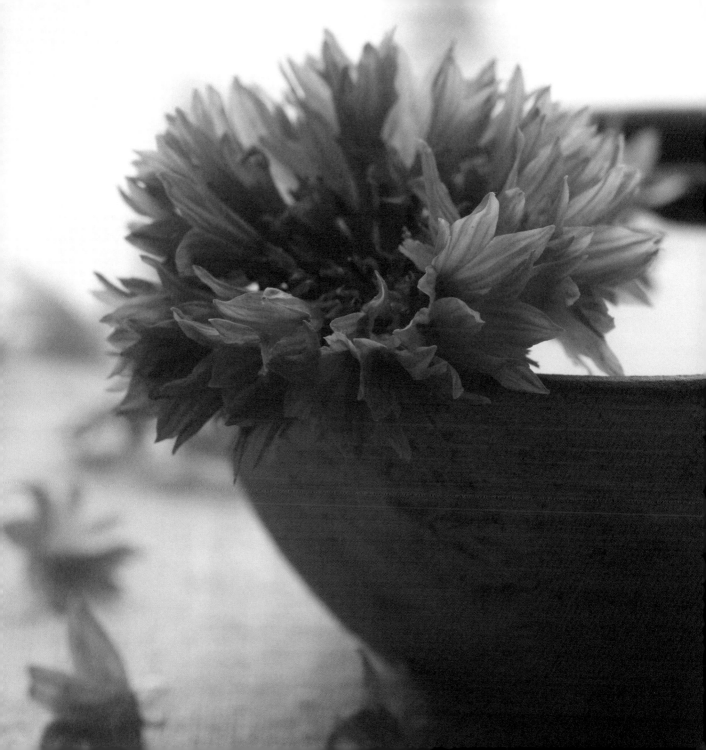

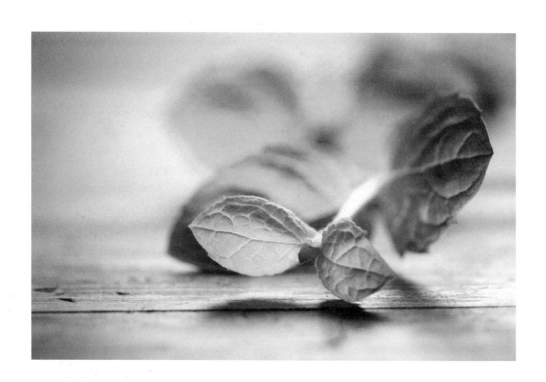

Combo Tea Eye Toner

The eyes quickly reveal symptoms of erratic sleep, too much time in front of the computer, or even a poor diet. Prepare this easy tea and herb blend, keep it handy, and use it to gently wipe tired eyelids twice a day for a fresher look.

INGREDIENTS

1 teaspoon chopped fresh mint leaves

1 teaspoon chopped fresh parsley leaves

1 chamomile tea bag

1 black tea bag

1 cup hot water

INSTRUCTIONS

1. Place the herbs and tea bag in a mug or small bowl, pour the water over them, cover, and allow 10 minutes steeping time.

2. Strain the liquid and transfer it to a bottle with a narrow opening. Close with a lid when the infusion has reached room temperature.

3. To use, soak a cotton ball, squeeze out excess liquid, and gently wipe (without pulling) tired eyelids twice a day.

4. Avoid getting any liquid in your eyes. Rinse with warm water if you like and pat dry.

5. Refrigerate any remainder and discard in a week.

Puffy Eyelids Compress

Sometimes the eyes need a little break. Plan a 15-minute time-out for your eyes once or twice a week, or whenever you feel that your tired puffy eyelids are begging for it. Potatoes have a skin-brightening effect and are rich in minerals (such as potassium) and enzymes (catecholase, in particular) that help reduce the puffiness of eyelids. Adding cucumber and black tea improves the results. Prepare this compress right before using it.

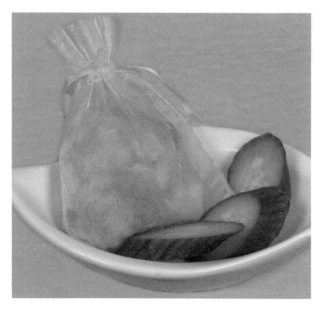

INGREDIENTS

- 2 tablespoons grated raw potato
- 2 tablespoons pureed cucumber
- 1 tablespoon black tea infusion (freshly prepared and cooled)
- 2 small organza bags

INSTRUCTIONS

1. In a small bowl, mix the ingredients well with a fork.

2. Pour half of the mixture into each organza bag. Let the excess liquid drain into the bowl before putting the bags on your eyelids.

3. Avoid getting any liquid in the eyes. Sit back and relax for 15 minutes. Rinse the eyes with warm water afterward and pat dry.

Anti-Aging Eye Cream

The very thin skin around the eyes is often the first to show signs of aging. This fragrance-free formula acts as a moisturizer and prevents premature signs of aging. While licorice extract has a skin-brightening effect that helps reduce the appearance of dark circles, evening primrose and wheat germ oils are sources of antioxidants and powerful anti-aging ingredients.

INGREDIENTS

- 1 teaspoon shea butter
- 1 teaspoon wheat germ oil
- 1 teaspoon evening primrose oil
- 1 teaspoon vegetable-derived emulsifier, such as glyceryl stearate
- 5 drops vitamin E
- 1 ounce (30 ml) rose water
- 2 drops rosemary oil extract
- 10 drops (0.5 ml) licorice extract

INSTRUCTIONS

1. Melt the shea butter in a double boiler over low heat, and then add the wheat germ and evening primrose oils and heat until the temperature reaches 170°F. Measure this using a candy thermometer. Add the emulsifier and whisk until completely dissolved. Add the vitamin E drops.

2. Simultaneously, gently heat the rose water in another double boiler, covering it with a lid to prevent evaporation. When both phases reach 170°F, turn off the heat and pour the oil phase, in a thin stream, into the water phase, whisking vigorously.

3. Keep on whisking until the creamy mixture is slightly warm (around 100°F).

4. Add the rosemary oil extract and the licorice extract, and keep whisking until completely blended.

5. Transfer the cream to a sanitized jar with a narrow opening and do not seal the lid until the mixture is no longer warm to the touch.

6. To use, dab small amounts of cream around the eye area morning and evening.

Anti-Aging Eye Balm

This formula is simple yet extremely nourishing; using it at bedtime brings antioxidants and moisture to the delicate wrinkle-prone skin of the eye area. Shea butter is a great moisturizer and can help transport other anti-aging oils such as sesame oil and cranberry oil. The addition of vitamin E will protect the oils from rancidity and increase its presence within the skin.

INGREDIENTS

1 ounce (30 ml) shea butter

1 teaspoon cranberry seed oil

1 teaspoon sesame oil

10 drops (0.5 ml) vitamin E oil

INSTRUCTIONS

1. In a double boiler, melt the shea butter over low heat without overheating. Whisk gently while adding the cranberry oil and sesame oil.

2. Add the vitamin E drops, then turn off the heat and continue whisking as you pour the mixture into a small tin box or glass jar.

3. Set aside to cool, and seal the lid when completely cool.

4. Apply in the evening by dabbing carefully around the eyes.

5. Store away from heat, light, and moisture.

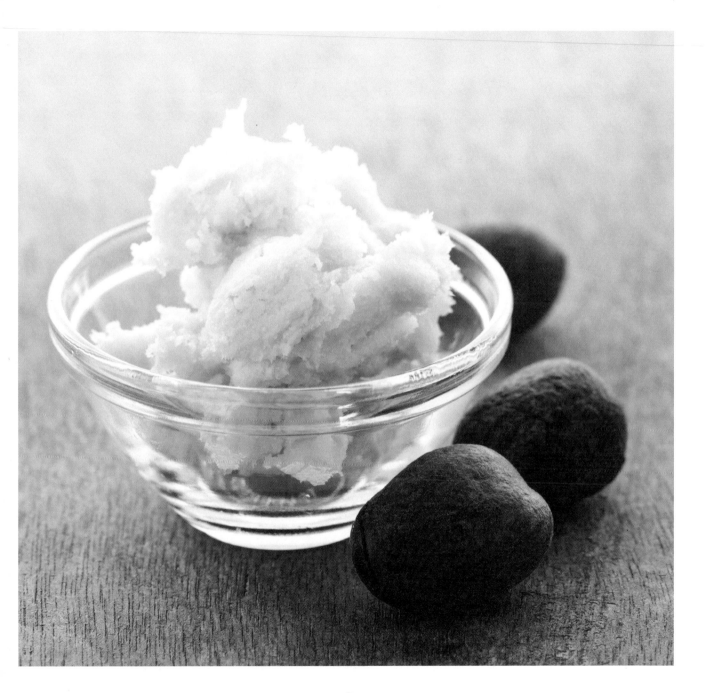

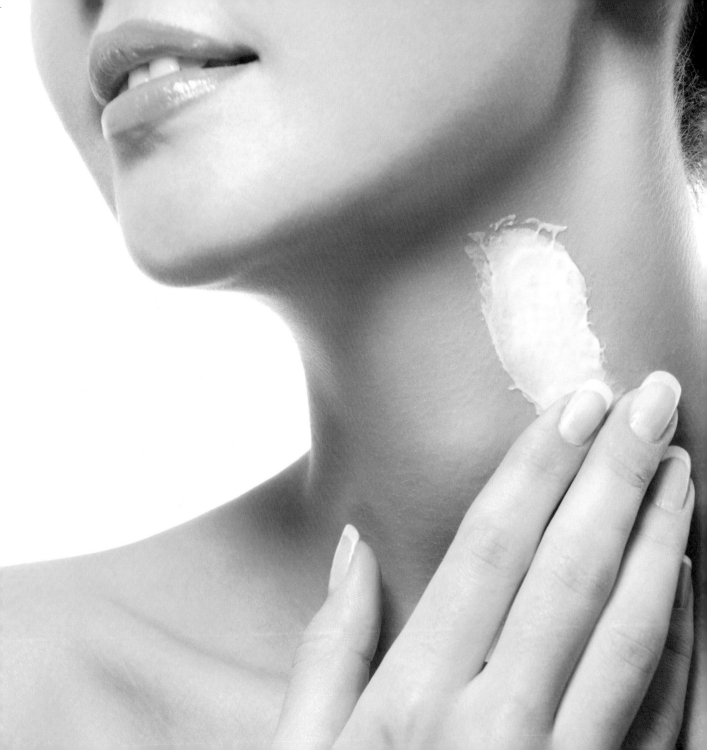

CHAPTER 11

Neck Care

The neck might be quick to reveal your true age. Weight loss, stress, a low-protein diet, and other reasons can lead to unappealing sagging, double chin, and wrinkles. It is, therefore, important to maintain a generous share of TLC for that specific area. Multiple recipes are provided in this chapter for you to choose from according to your own needs.

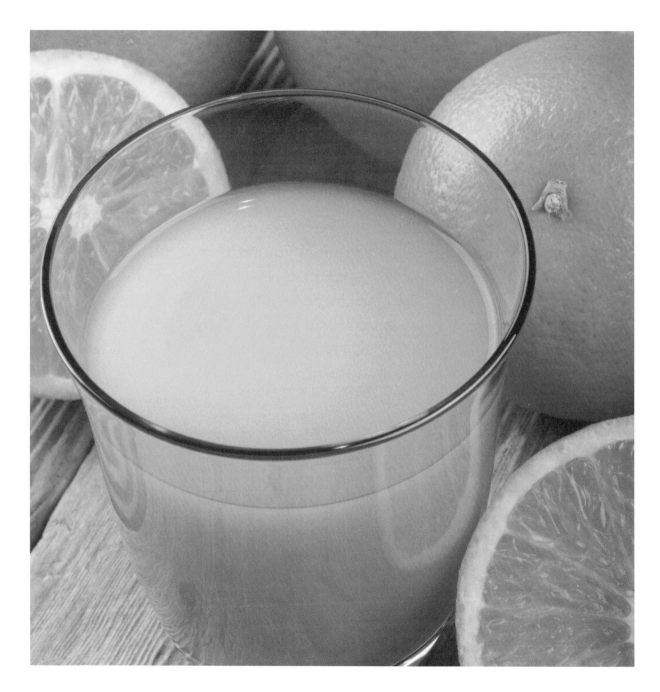

Moisturizer Plus Mask

We all know that the neck deserves a daily share of the facial moisturizer. However, we sometimes feel that we need a little extra lifting and tightening of that skin. Because of their high protein content, egg whites offer a skin-tightening effect, while egg yolks supplement the skin with cholesterol and unsaturated fats. Vitamin C, from orange juice, will help rejuvenate the skin and fight aging; vitamin E will allow for the antioxidant effect of vitamin C and provide a wrinkle-fighting effect. Just a little cologne is added to improve the fragrance. Once prepared, you can store this mask in the refrigerator for up to a week.

INGREDIENTS

1 egg
1 teaspoon freshly squeezed orange juice
10 drops (0.5 ml) baby cologne
5 drops (0.5 ml) vitamin E
4 teaspoons (20 ml) of your usual daily moisturizer

INSTRUCTIONS

1. Beat the egg and continue beating it as you slowly add the juice, cologne, and vitamin E.

2. Pour the egg mixture over the moisturizing cream gradually and in a very thin stream, whipping vigorously to incorporate.

3. Transfer the mixture to a pump bottle and apply like a lotion. Wait for 10 minutes before rinsing with water; then using your usual cleanser. Follow with your moisturizer. Apply twice a day, over a week, to tone the skin.

4. Store the mask in the refrigerator for no longer than a week.

Extra-Nourishing Neck Care

This mask has virtually all the nutrients that skin could lack. Use it once a week on the neck to tighten, brighten, firm, and rewind age.

INGREDIENTS

2 cups (500 ml) freshly made linden tea

1 egg yolk

1 medium-size potato, cooked and mashed

1 tablespoon royal jelly

1 teaspoon lemon juice

1 tablespoon almond oil

5 drops vitamin E

gauze strips

Note: You can substitute honey for the royal jelly, according to availability.

INSTRUCTIONS

1. Start by preparing 2 cups of linden tea (1 teaspoon per cup of water), and set it aside to cool. Add the egg yolk to the mashed potato. Mix well until completely blended. Pour the royal jelly over the mixture and blend again. Finish by adding the lemon juice, almond oil, and vitamin E.

2. Put the mixture in the refrigerator to chill. Meanwhile, prepare rectangular gauze sheets in double layers, making sure they will easily cover and wrap around the neck and under the chin.

3. Spread the chilled mixture on gauze strips and apply directly to your neck and under your chin. Sit back and relax for 15–20 minutes.

4. Remove the mask and wash your skin with the lukewarm linden tea. Follow with a facial moisturizer.

5. Use this mask weekly over a three-month period for better-lasting effects.

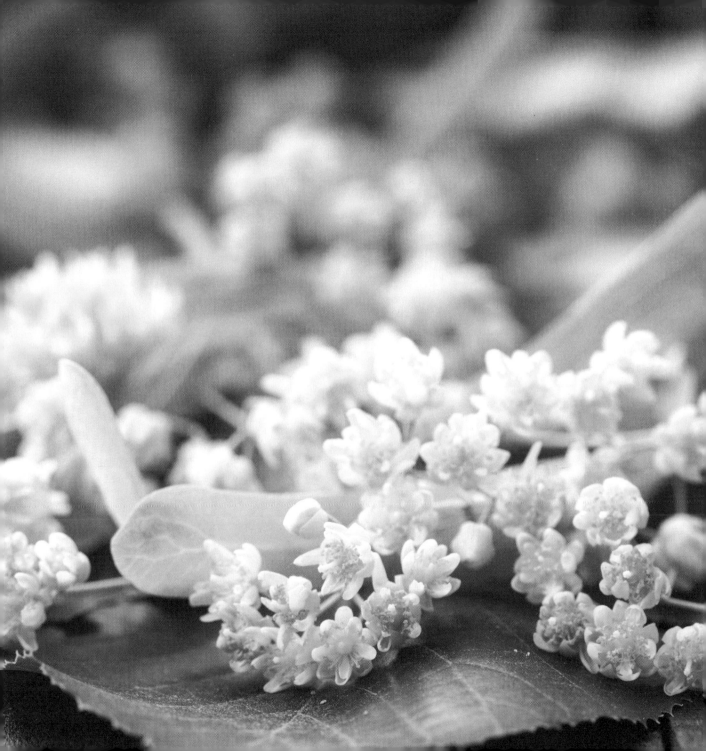

Biweekly Neck Lift Mask

This formula will improve the skin's elasticity. The acidity of the yogurt will help get rid of old skin cells, while the avocado oil nourishes the skin with essential fatty acids and generous amounts of vitamin E. Borage seed oil prevents wrinkles, and vitamin C rejuvenates the skin.

INGREDIENTS

1 tablespoon avocado oil

1 medium-size potato, cooked and mashed

2 ounces (60 ml) full-fat plain yogurt (preferably organic)

1 tablespoon orange juice

1 teaspoon borage seed oil

gauze strips

INSTRUCTIONS

1. Pour the avocado oil over the mashed potato and mix well until absorbed. Add the yogurt and orange juice and mix again. Finish by blending in the borage seed oil.

2. Cover and refrigerate for 20–30 minutes. Meanwhile, prepare your gauze strips. Cut generous double layers of gauze in rectangles. Make sure the strips will cover your neck and under the chin area. Allow extra length to wrap around the neck.

3. Remove the mixture from the refrigerator and spread it like sandwich filling between the layers of gauze.

4. Wash your neck with warm water, dry with a towel, and then apply the gauze pads. Sit back and relax for 10 minutes. Flip the gauze strips to renew contact and relax for another 10 minutes. Remove the gauze and rinse the area. Follow with your daily moisturizer.

5. Use any leftovers three days later, and try to use this mask twice weekly for three months for most sustainable results.

Neck Tight and Bright Serum

This egg-based serum has wonderful effects on the skin, especially when used regularly in combination with one of the previous neck masks. It is easy to make and has a high protein content that can help tighten skin.

INGREDIENTS

2 egg whites

1 teaspoon lemon juice

1 ounce (30 ml) aloe vera gel

1 teaspoon avocado oil

INSTRUCTIONS

1. Whisk the egg whites and lemon juice together; then add the aloe vera gel and whisk again. Use a stick blender if you like. Pour the avocado oil very slowly into the mixture, continuing to whisk until completely blended.

2. Transfer the mixture to a pump bottle, and always shake the bottle before pumping.

3. Spread on your neck and under the chin area every evening. Allow at least 20 minutes contact time before rinsing, or rinse the following morning. Follow with a moisturizer and sunscreen.

4. Store this mixture in the refrigerator for up to a week.

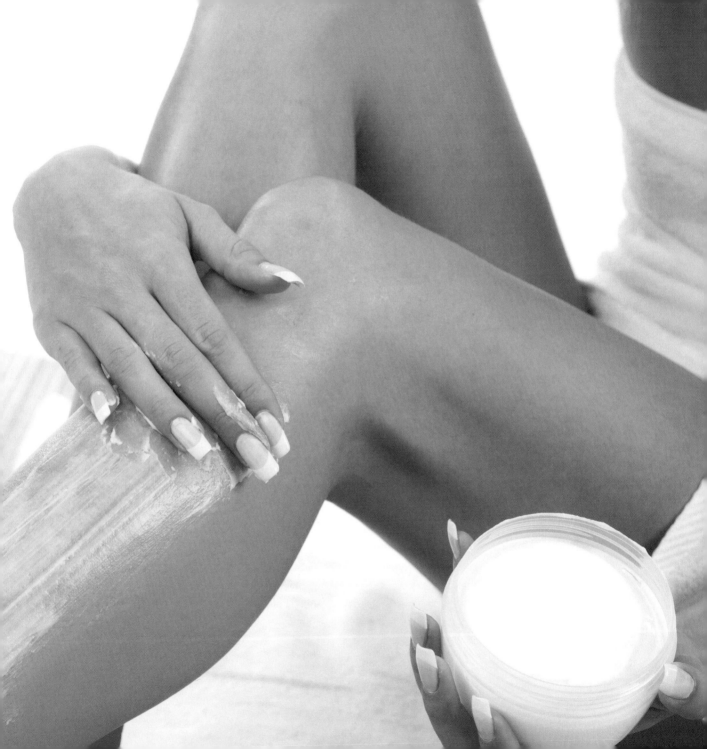

CHAPTER 12

Body Care

The skin of the body needs as much special care as the face does, as it is subject to weather aggression, weight changes, waxing, shaving, and loss of water from summer sweating. Keeping it moisturized, soft, and nourished is important to maintain good skin tone and feel.

Yummy Body Scrub

Though it's a little rough on facial skin, brown sugar makes an excellent body scrub. Vanilla and rose water contribute to making a nicely scented formula. The addition of olive oil, which is a great long-lasting moisturizer, guarantees that this formula will leave dry skin feeling softened and velvety.

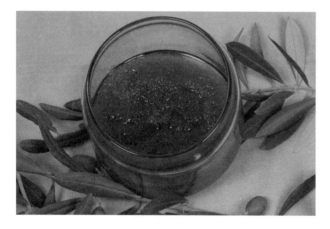

INGREDIENTS

1 cup brown sugar

3 ounces (100 ml) olive oil

3 ounces (100 ml) sunflower oil

1 tablespoon rose water

20 drops (1 ml) vanilla extract

INSTRUCTIONS

1. Combine all ingredients in their listed order and mix well, making sure the sugar is "soaked" with oil.

2. Transfer to a wide-mouth plastic container.

3. Right before you finish showering, dip your fingertips in the jar, take out some of the mix and rub in circular motions onto your body, mainly legs and arms, to help get rid of dead skin cells.

4. Rinse off with warm water and pat yourself dry.

5. Cover the jar and save the remainder for subsequent use.

Honey Oatmeal Scrub

This scrub combines the moisturizing effects of ground oats and aloe vera with the anti-aging properties of honey for much more than simple exfoliation.

Oatmeal is rich in vitamin E; mixed with almond meal, it gives this scrub a rougher texture that will help get rid of dead skin cells. Honey is also a humectant, which retains moisture. Apricot kernel oil will moisturize and soften the skin for a silky after-feel. Use this mask once a week, especially during harsh winter months.

INGREDIENTS

1 ounce (30 ml) honey

½ cup almond meal

½ cup ground oats

1 cup aloe vera gel

1 ounce (30 ml) apricot kernel oil

INSTRUCTIONS

1. Mix the honey with 1 ounce of the almond meal; then mix the remaining almond meal with the ground oats. Drizzle apricot kernel oil into the honey–almond meal blend, and mix again, incorporating the almont meal-ground oats mixture. Gradually add the aloe vera gel, mixing well to avoid lumps.

2. Transfer the mixture to a wide-mouth plastic container.

3. At the end of your shower, rub this mix on your body in circular motions to exfoliate the skin. Rinse off with plenty of water.

Fragrant Body Mask

The following formula is something between a mask and a lotion. It is greatly moisturizing because of the creaminess of half-and-half, which will boost the skin's lipid barrier, while honey and glycerin will draw moisture to it. Rose water will leave a soft flowery scent all over the body, and vitamin E is an antioxidant and an anti-aging ingredient that will perfect the efficacy of the mix.

INGREDIENTS

1 tablespoon honey

2 ounces (60 ml) rose water

1 tablespoon vegetable-derived glycerin

½ cup half-and-half

20 drops (1 ml) vitamin E

INSTRUCTIONS

1. Dissolve the honey in the rose water; then add the glycerin and the half-and-half. Add the vitamin E, whisk, and then pour all ingredients into a bottle. Seal tightly and shake vigorously.

2. Refrigerate this mixture until you are ready for it. Use in a day or two at the latest.

3. At the end of your shower, pour small amounts in your palms and spread on legs and arms.

4. Wait a few minutes, then rinse with warm water, and pat your body dry with a towel.

Fragrant Body Balm

Balms are oils, butters, and waxes with insignificant water content.
Apply balms on dry body areas directly after showering, when the skin is still moist, making sure to rub generously on knees, elbows, and heels. One major advantage of balms over creams and lotions is the extended shelf life. Because of their lack of water, they are less favorable for bacterial growth. Proper storage aims at avoiding heat, light, and humidity, to preserve the oils and protect them from rancidity.

INGREDIENTS

1 teaspoon grated beeswax

1 ounce (30 ml) shea butter

1 ounce (30 ml) apricot kernel oil

1 ounce (30 ml) jojoba oil

10 drops (0.5 ml) grapefruit essential oil

INSTRUCTIONS

1. Melt the beeswax and butter in a double boiler over low heat. Add the apricot kernel and jojoba oils in a thin stream, one at a time, whisking continuously.

2. Turn off the heat and add the grapefruit essential oil before the mixture starts to solidify. When thoroughly blended, transfer the mixture to a glass jar or a tin box. Allow the balm to reach room temperature before putting the lid on.

3. Rub quarter-size amounts on dry areas of the body, preferably after showering, to retain moisture.

Winter Balm

This is every family's must-have balm during harsh winters. Super easy to make, wonderfully scented, and multipurpose, it can be prepared during the fall and kept handy to rescue those frequently chapped areas: elbows, knees, lips, hands, and heels.

INGREDIENTS

1 tablespoon grated beeswax (or beeswax pellets)

2 ounces (60 ml) almond oil

1 tablespoon vegetable-derived glycerin

20 drops (1 ml) vanilla essence or lavender essential oil

20 drops (1 ml) vitamin E oil

INSTRUCTIONS

1. Use a double boiler to melt the beeswax. Add the almond oil and stir to mix. Add the glycerin, vanilla, and vitamin E. Stir well.

2. Pour into small tin containers. Allow the balm to cool before sealing the lids.

3. Keep handy and use just like any other balm.

Spicy Body Oil

This formula makes a moisturizing yet light body oil that can also be used as a pleasant-smelling massage oil. It is most suitable for winter because of its texture and warm scent.

INGREDIENTS

2 ounces (60 ml) almond oil

2 ounces (60 ml) jojoba oil

2 ounces (60 ml) sunflower oil

3 large cinnamon sticks

7–8 cloves

1 teaspoon freshly grated nutmeg

20 drops (1 ml) vanilla essential oil

20 drops (1 ml) vitamin E

2 small organza bags

INSTRUCTIONS

1. Combine the three oils and transfer to a jar.

2. Break the cinnamon sticks into small pieces and drop them into the oils. Throw in the cloves. Pour ½ teaspoon nutmeg into one small organza bag and another ½ teaspoon into the other bag, and drop them both into the mix.

3. Stir well to make sure the spices are soaked with the oils; then cover the jar with a lid and set aside, away from light and heat. Shake the jar multiple times daily to promote transfer of the oils.

4. After a week, remove the cinnamon sticks and cloves and squeeze the organza bags before removing them, as well.

5. Add the vanilla essential oil and vitamin E and stir.

6. Pour the scented oil into an amber bottle to minimize oxidation. Use as a gender-neutral body oil.

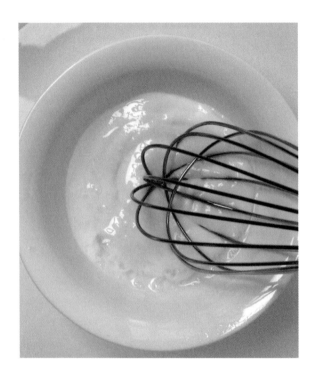

Fragrant Body Lotion

This formula is an excellent moisturizer that leaves skin feeling soft, wonderfully scented, and nourished, with no greasy after-feel.

INGREDIENTS

½ cup daily moisturizing cream

1 ounce (30 ml) orange blossom water (neroli hydrosol)

5 drops grapefruit essential oil

INSTRUCTIONS

1. You will need two double boilers: one to warm up your daily moisturizer and another one for the flower water. It is important that the two ingredients reach similar temperatures (usually 160–180°F) for best mixability. Measure this using a candy thermometer.

2. Once this has been achieved, turn off the heat, and pour the neroli water in a very thin stream over the cream, whisking vigorously (use a stick blender if available and watch out for splashes).

3. Allow the mixture to cool before adding the essential oil. Mix again, then pour into a pump bottle. Use more flower water for a thinner texture, or more cream for a thicker texture.

4. Apply once or twice daily as a body moisturizer. Avoid sun exposure to prevent photosensitivity.

Mediterranean Body Polish

Very easy to make and to apply, with wonderful, lasting results, this simple formula is a busy mom's best friend, especially during winter when the skin needs a lot of TLC and little time is available. Olive oil will leave skin feeling softer and better moisturized for the following day. The addition of an essential oil will make this body oil pleasant to the senses.

INGREDIENTS

½ cup extra virgin olive oil

½ cup almond oil

½ cup grape seed oil

20 drops (1 ml) vitamin E

20 drops (1 ml) Rosa damascena essential oil (or another more affordable essential oil of your choice, such as gardenia or geranium)

INSTRUCTIONS

1. Mix all the above ingredients together and transfer the mixture to a pump bottle.

2. Before stepping out of the shower, while your body is still wet, pump a little oil into the palm of your hands and spread it on your legs and arms. Dry yourself with a towel, as usual.

3. Use daily or as often as time allows, for silky soft skin.

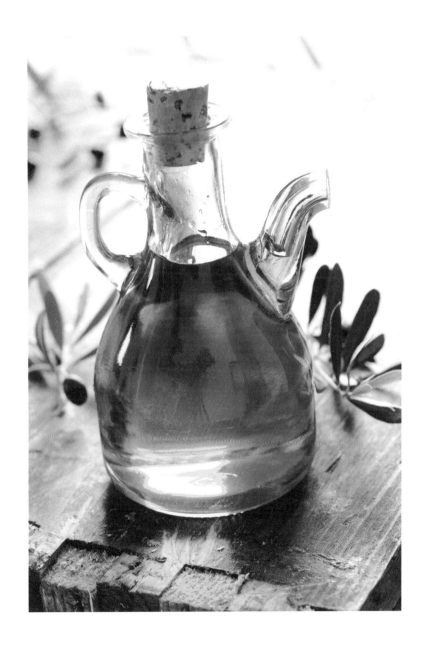

Relaxation Massage Oil

This is a simple and calming massage oil that brings moisture, softness, and vitamin E to the skin. The chosen oils spread easily and do not clog pores, while ylang-ylang helps you unwind.

INGREDIENTS

- 2 ounces (60 ml) almond oil
- 2 ounces (60 ml) sunflower oil
- 2 ounces (60 ml) jojoba oil
- 20 drops (1 ml) ylang-ylang essential oil (or your own favorite blend)

INSTRUCTIONS

1. Transfer the ingredients one at a time to an amber glass bottle. Always leave essential oils for the last step to prevent their evaporation.

2. Shake well and use as a regular massage oil.

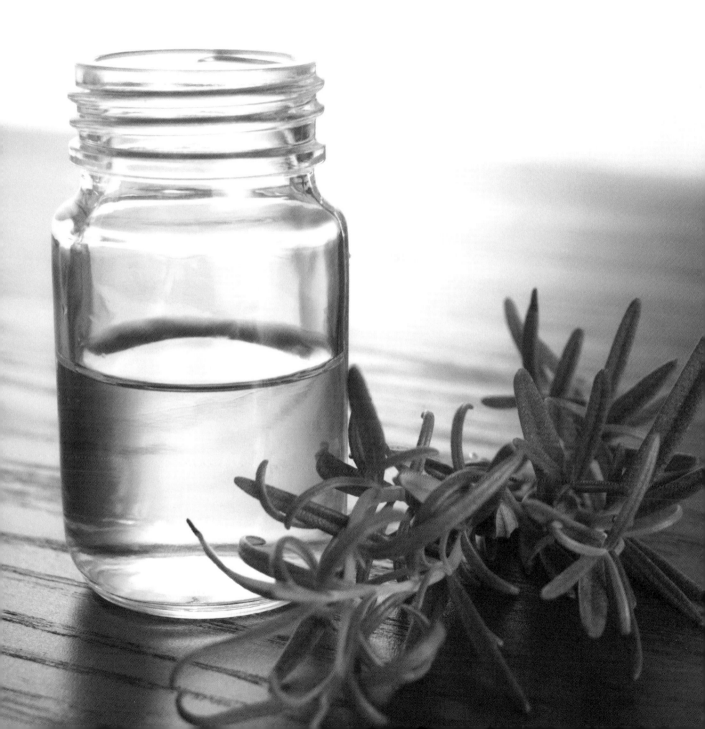

Refreshing Body Gel

Big summer favorites, gels are extremely rich in water. While this gel may look like thickened water, other elements give it specific properties that water alone cannot provide: mint and peppermint are highly refreshing and cooling, and alfalfa is rejuvenating. Enjoy this gel during summer at the end of a day on the beach.

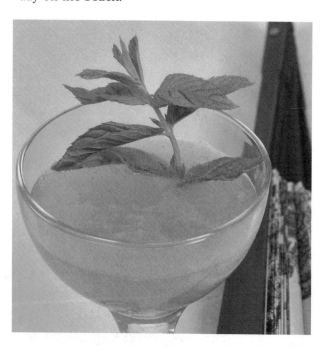

INGREDIENTS

2 ounces (60 ml) purified water

2 ounces (60 ml) mint infusion

¼ teaspoon alfalfa extract

10 drops (0.5 ml) peppermint essential oil (optional)

¼ teaspoon xanthan gum

Note: You can substitute aloe vera gel for the water to facilitate gel formation.

INSTRUCTIONS

1. Mix the water and mint infusion and bring the temperature of the mixture to a warm range of 100°F by heating over a direct flame. Measure this using a candy thermometer.

2. Add the alfalfa extract and then the peppermint essential oil, whisking well to disperse.

3. Whisk while gently sprinkling the xanthan gum over the surface of the water mixture. Avoid using too much, because it might make your gel stringy and slimy, with an unpleasant texture. Eliminate any lumps; use a stick blender if needed. Transfer the mixture to a bottle.

4. Use this gel on hot days, after being in the sun—or after hair removal—to soothe and refresh the skin.

Smooth-and-Shiny-Legs Scrub

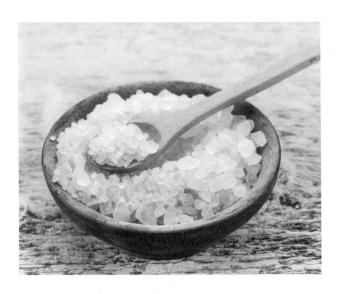

This formula makes a great mask to improve the appearance of arms and legs. Almond meal and Himalayan salt are exfoliating agents that will help renew skin and diminish ingrown hair. Olive oil and honey make this mask highly moisturizing, and lemon juice brings generous amounts of vitamin C to smooth skin and counteract any discoloration.

INGREDIENTS

1 ounce (30 ml) honey

2 teaspoons lemon juice

2 ounces (60 ml) olive oil

1 teaspoon sea salt or Himalayan pink salt

1 ounce (30 ml) almond meal

INSTRUCTIONS

1. In a bowl, using a small whisk, mix the honey with the lemon juice; then add the olive oil.

2. Separately, mix the salt with the almond meal, and gradually add to the liquid mixture.

3. At the end of your shower, when your skin is still wet and ready for exfoliation, spread the mixture on your legs (and arms, if you like) and wait 5–10 minutes.

4. Remove by scrubbing, focusing on ingrown hair zones. Rinse off with warm water and pat your body dry with a towel. Avoid sun exposure to prevent photosensitivity.

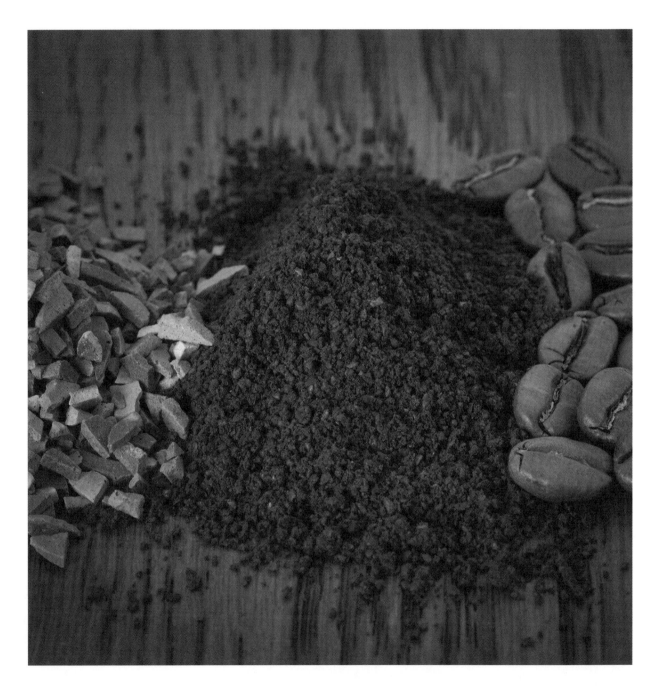

Anti-Cellulite Body Wrap

While many people think of cellulite as fat deposits, specialists look at it as a sign of poor drainage of water and toxins. What causes cellulite formation? The answer to this question is complex, especially when we consider that men and women, adults and children, lean and overweight people, can have cellulite. It is recommended to avoid tight-fitting clothes that compress vessels and tissues and prevent adequate drainage, to drink a lot of water to enhance drainage, and to massage trouble areas to improve skin texture.

Alongside these measures, the diuretic effects of caffeine masks are helpful in decreasing retention of water under the skin.

However, keep in mind that caffeine can be absorbed through the skin. Do not use if you are pregnant or nursing. If you cannot tolerate strong coffee, this formula may not be for you. If you have high blood pressure, fast heart rate, arrhythmias, kidney disease, or other medical conditions, check with your doctor first.

Sea kelp is incorporated into this formula to enhance the effect of caffeine. It is rich in silica, which helps with skin regeneration. Any caffeinated coffee grounds (coarse or fine) are okay to use in this formula. Flavored coffee (hazelnut, vanilla, or other) will make a nicer-smelling mask.

INGREDIENTS

1 cup caffeinated coffee grounds
½ cup sea kelp powder
½–1 cup aloe vera gel
5–10 drops vanilla extract (optional)

INSTRUCTIONS

1. Begin by mixing the coffee grounds with the sea kelp powder. Use enough aloe vera gel to bind the coffee grounds and sea kelp powder and achieve a consistency you can work with. Add vanilla extract, if using.

2. Spread the mixture on plastic film and wrap the film around your thighs with the mixture on the inside. Leave on for 15 minutes. Then remove the wrap and rinse your skin.

3. Repeat twice a week for up to 12 weeks for optimal results.

Hair Removal Sugar Paste

Extremely common and widely used around the world, this natural recipe is easy to prepare and is very economical. Sugar paste is among the safest depilatory methods. The pain generated when the hair is pulled from follicles is similar to that generated during waxing except that no strips are needed. Sugar paste will also remove dead cells and help renew the epithelium (the skin surface). That is why you can expect fewer ingrown hairs than with electric epilators. Prepare a generous quantity, divide it in half, and store the extra paste in the refrigerator for future use. Keep away from children.

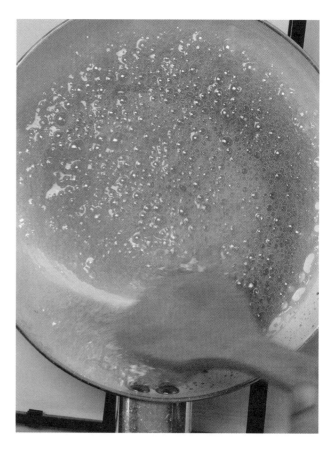

INGREDIENTS

1½ cups sugar

1 cup water

1 teaspoon lemon juice

INSTRUCTIONS

1. Pour the sugar into a saucepan. Drizzle the water over it and place the pan over medium heat, stirring with a wooden spoon. The initial cloudiness of the sugar will gradually disappear as more sugar particles dissolve in the hot water. Continue stirring even when the mixture starts to boil and bubbles form.

2. Add the lemon juice while maintaining the medium heat.

3. Watch the color of the bubbling liquid at the edge of the pan. When golden bubbles start to form at the edge, stir a little more until all the liquid is golden.

4. Do not overcook the sugar, because that will transform it into hard candy.

5. Turn off the heat and pour the sugar paste into a wide-mouth glass jar.

6. When it starts to cool down, use a tablespoon to scoop out some sugar paste. Now it's Play-Doh time. Roll the paste into a ball, then stretch and fold the paste on itself a few times to soften it, moistening your fingers if needed. The paste is ready to use when it stretches easily and doesn't stick to your fingers.

7. Your skin needs to be clean, dry, and free from lotions and oils. With your thumbs, press firmly as you spread the paste in the opposite direction of the hair growth. Flick it sharply backward to remove. Repeat on other skin sections until all area hair is removed.

8. Wash your skin under warm water. No oils are needed to remove traces of sugar paste, since it dissolves in water.

9. Follow with a refreshing gel to soothe the skin. Store the unused sugar paste in the refrigerator for later use. Soften it when needed using a double boiler or microwave.

Anti-Stretchmark Balm

During pregnancy, the breasts and belly increase in size, which forces the skin to stretch accordingly. Overall weight gain is also a reason for significant stretching. This challenges the skin's elasticity, and stretch marks may appear.

It is much easier to prevent stretch marks than to treat them, and prevention is recommended as early as possible during pregnancy, even before. This formula uses simple and organic ingredients without any added fragrance that pregnant women may not tolerate. It contains no water and stores well.

INGREDIENTS

2 ounces (60 ml) organic cocoa butter

1 tablespoon organic almond oil

1 tablespoon cucumber seed oil

10 drops (0.5 ml) vitamin E

Note: You can substitute shea butter for the cocoa butter and olive oil for the cucumber seed oil, depending on availability, nut allergies, and scent tolerance.

INSTRUCTIONS

1. Melt the cocoa butter in a double boiler, over low heat; then add the almond and cucumber seed oils. Whisk until well blended and then remove from the heat. Continue whisking as the mixture cools.

2. Pour the mixture into a dark glass jar with a wide mouth, and set aside. Seal with a lid when completely cooled.

3. Rub on your belly, or other part of your body, twice daily, preferably after showering.

4. Store away from heat and humidity.

Anti-Stretchmark Oil

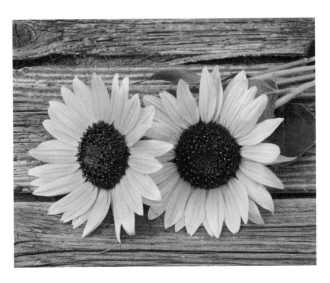

INGREDIENTS

3 ounces (100 ml) sunflower oil

1 ounce (30 ml) grape seed oil

1 ounce (30 ml) olive oil

20 (1 ml) drops vitamin E

5 drops lavender essential oil (optional)

Note: You can substitute wheat germ oil or rice bran oil for the olive oil to eliminate that scent if morning sickness makes it bothersome to your senses.

INSTRUCTIONS

1. Pour all the ingredients into a bowl and whisk to mix thoroughly; then transfer to an amber bottle.

2. Apply daily to wet skin after showering.

3. Store away from heat, light, and humidity.

This is a simple and easy way to make an unscented oil that can be quickly spread all over the body, belly included, to prevent stretch marks. It is rich in natural vitamin E and unsaturated fatty acids that improve skin elasticity. This formula does not call for almond oil, so is safe to use in case of a nut allergy. It is safe to use during pregnancy and while breastfeeding. Use food-grade, preferably organic, oils when they're available.

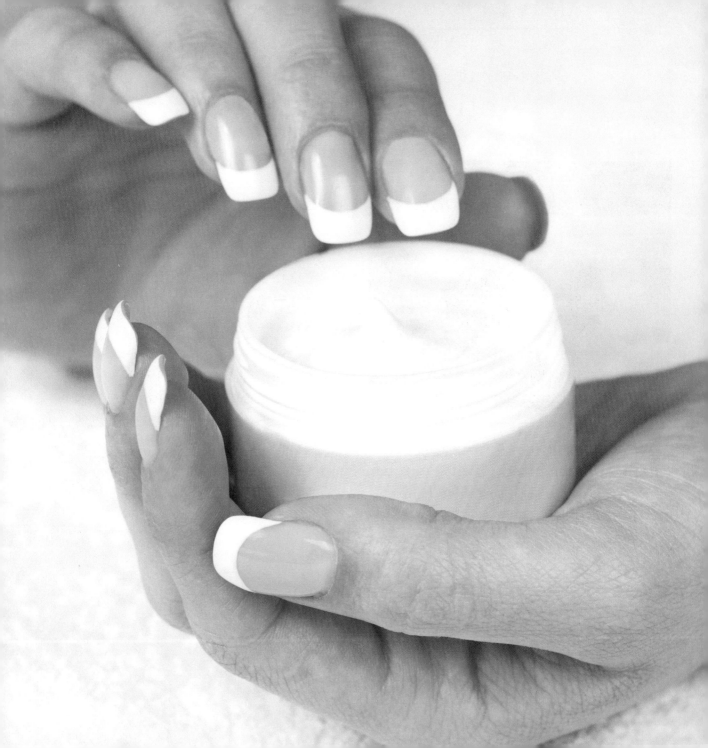

CHAPTER 13

Hand Care

Hands can often give away age, even before little wrinkles around eyes and lips appear. The skin on top of the hands is thin, with small muscles and little fat to support it. Also, it is rarely covered and is therefore exposed to virtually all kinds of weather, as well as soap and water and potentially harsh detergents. During winter, hands become dry and chapped. In summer, most hands get more sun than the rest of the body. For all these reasons, our hands may not look their best and may require special attention.

Double-Agent Hand Mask

This mask begins with an exfoliating phase that will take off all the dryness on top of your hands and prepare newer skin cells for a makeover. The second phase combines the firming effect of egg whites with the nutritious properties of honey. Cream cheese provides a fat component that will soften the skin.

INGREDIENTS FOR PHASE 1

½ cup semolina

1 teaspoon sea salt

1 ounce (30 ml) olive oil

2 ounces (60 ml) almond milk

INSTRUCTIONS

1. Mix all the above ingredients.

2. Apply by rubbing on the hands with circular motions for a couple of minutes. Make sure to rub around the fingernails, as well, to improve cuticle appearance. Then rinse off. Repeat one more time.

3. You should be able to tell the difference by feeling smoother skin on your hands.

INGREDIENTS FOR PHASE 2

1 tablespoon softened cream cheese

1 tablespoon honey

1 egg

Disposable gloves

Note: If you are allergic to eggs, replace the egg with 1 tablespoon olive oil.

INSTRUCTIONS

1. Mix the cream cheese and honey, and set the mixture aside. Whisk the egg; then add it to the creamy mixture.

2. Spread the mixture on your hands, and then put on the disposable gloves. Wait 10–15 minutes before removing the gloves and washing your hands.

3. Follow with your usual hand cream.

Youthful Hand Concoction

Hands age as fast as the face, sometimes even faster, and people may be able to guess your age only by looking at your hands. This formula combines essential elements and a few extra proteins to help hands fight aging, reverse sun damage, and remain soft to the touch.

INGREDIENTS

1 egg white
1 ounce (30 ml) heavy cream
½ teaspoon lemon juice
2 teaspoons almond oil

INSTRUCTIONS

1. Whisk together all the above ingredients in their listed order and transfer the mixture to a bottle.

2. Rub a little on both hands twice a day. Leave on for 10–15 minutes before washing. Follow with a sunscreen in the morning, especially if your hands will be exposed to sunlight.

3. Store in the refrigerator for up to a week. Shake well before each application.

Weather Shield Mask

This mask is good in wintertime, when hands tend to become dry and rough. Prepare as often as needed to whiten and nourish hands.

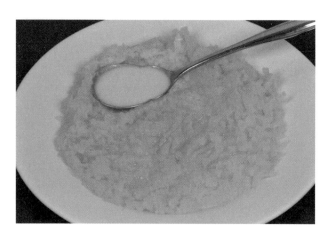

INGREDIENTS

4 small potatoes, peeled, cooked, and mashed

1 ounce (30 ml) heavy cream

1 tablespoon olive oil

1 tablespoon lemon juice

10 drops (0.5 ml) vitamin E

INSTRUCTIONS

1. Mix the above ingredients well until a uniform paste is formed.

2. Spread the mask on your hands and rub in well to help the fats from the cream and oil penetrate the skin.

3. Keep this mask on for a few minutes; then rinse off with warm water. Follow with a hand moisturizer.

Round-the-Clock Hand Moisturizer

As its name suggests, this silky moisturizer can be used as many times as needed during the day. Prepare this moisturizer as often as you like and store it in a pump bottle right next to your hand soap.

INGREDIENTS

4 ounces (60 ml) aloe vera gel

2 teaspoons almond oil

1 teaspoon vegetable-derived glycerin

INSTRUCTIONS

1. Start with the gel, to which you will add the almond oil, 1 teaspoon at a time, whisking continuously. Add the glycerin, whisk well for several minutes, and then transfer to a pump bottle.

2. Apply as often as your hands need it, especially after washing with soap or working with detergents.

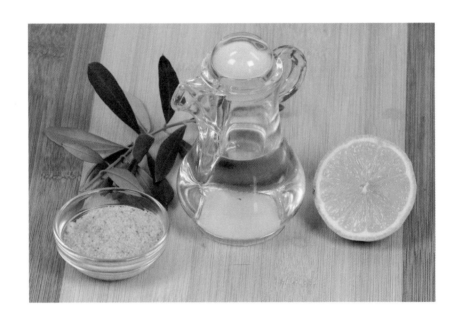

Hand and Elbow Formula

This extremely simple recipe may look like a Mediterranean salad dressing, but it's much more than that. Olive oil is a wonderful moisturizer, and lemon juice will brighten your hands and elbows. Himalayan salt contains more than 80 minerals and helps with exfoliation. Prepare frequently to soften rough areas on the hands and elbows.

INGREDIENTS

2 ounces (60 ml) extra virgin olive oil

2 ounces (60 ml) sunflower oil

1 ounce (30 ml) lemon juice

1 pinch Himalayan salt

INSTRUCTIONS

1. Mix the oils together, then whisk in the lemon juice. Sprinkle the salt in gradually and whisk continuously to blend. Use a stick blender to achieve better mixing.

2. Transfer the mixture to a bottle. Always shake vigorously before applying to hands and elbows. Follow with sunscreen prior to sun exposure.

Soft and Bright Hands

This recipe calls for a few drops of white vinegar, which acts as a keratolytic (remover of dead skin cells) and a skin brightener capable of revealing newer skin. Prepare this formula if you need to improve the appearance of sunspots on your hands. The addition of more friendly ingredients will compensate for the harsh acidity and drying effect of the vinegar.

INGREDIENTS

- 2 ounces (60 ml) rose water
- 2 ounces (60 ml) pulp-free cucumber juice
- 1 tablespoon vegetable-derived glycerin
- 1 tablespoon white vinegar (5% acidity)

INSTRUCTIONS

1. Combine the rose water with the cucumber juice in a small bowl. Then, stirring continuously, slowly pour the glycerin into the rose water and cucumber juice. Add the white vinegar, mix, and transfer to a bottle.

2. Spread a small amount on the hands once daily, preferably at bedtime. Alternate with a hand moisturizer and a sunscreen in the morning.

All-Natural Hand Sanitizer

Rubbing alcohol is a widely used sanitizer with reliable efficacy.
The U.S. Food and Drug Administration (FDA) recommends a concentration ranging from 60 percent to 95 percent ethanol or isopropanol for effective germicidal activity.

Once you try this recipe, you will stop buying commercial hand sanitizers. It is so easy to make and costs a fraction of the price. You can prepare enough for a whole season and refill small empty spray bottles as you go.

The formula has three basic ingredients:

- The sanitizing agent: rubbing alcohol. Rubbing alcohol is not pure alcohol. It is diluted with water to a 70 percent concentration. Make sure you use a reputable brand because alcohol can carry many impurities that you do not want.

- Essential oils (such as thyme or eucalyptus oils) help improve the smell of the spray and may provide antiseptic properties of their own.

- Glycerin or aloe vera will counterbalance the drying effect of the rubbing alcohol on the skin.

INGREDIENTS

3 ounces (100 ml) 70 percent rubbing alcohol
1 teaspoon vegetable-derived glycerin
1 teaspoon aloe vera juice
20 drops (1 ml) thyme (or other) essential oil

INSTRUCTIONS

1. Mix all the above ingredients and transfer the mixture to a spray bottle.

2. Use to sanitize hands when needed.

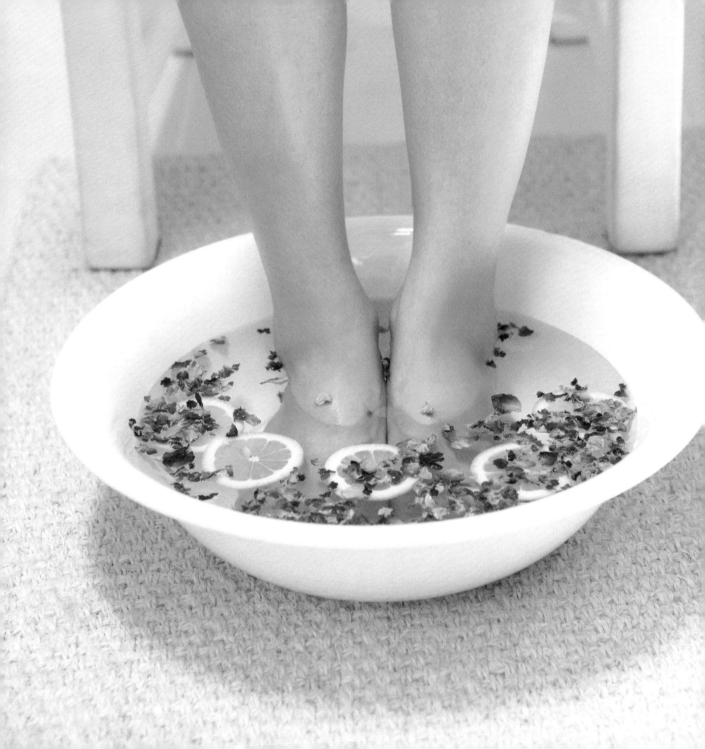

CHAPTER 14

Foot and Heel Care

Even though the feet are not usually as exposed as the face and hands, they do need an equivalent amount of TLC. The most common problems are dry, cracked heels and foot odor. The simple, effective, and inexpensive fixes in this chapter can solve those issues in no time.

Lemon Peel Quick Fix

The following recipe may be one of the easiest, fastest, and funniest fixes for your heels. Lemons are rich in vitamin C, and the acidity retained in the peel or rind helps with dead cell exfoliation.

The regular use of a pumice stone during your shower is highly recommended.

INGREDIENTS

1 large lemon cut in half

2 teaspoons olive oil

2 pairs spa or winter socks (soft & plush, non-cotton)

INSTRUCTIONS

1. Squeeze the juice out of the lemons and set it aside for another use. Place the white inside of a rind against each heel, using bandages if needed to hold the rinds in place against your heels.

2. Pull socks on over the rinds and keep them on for half an hour.

3. Remove your socks and the lemon rinds and massage 1 teaspoon of olive oil into each foot, especially the heels. Put on another pair of socks for another 30 minutes to soften the heels further.

Foot Soak

Prepare this recipe at the end of a long day. Soak your feet to relax, get rid of odor, and improve blood circulation. While ginger stimulates circulation, rosemary relieves inflammation, mint takes away odors, and tea tree oil helps kill bacteria. There is a small quantity of grape seed oil to soften and nourish the feet.

See How to Make Your Own Infusions, Decoctions, and Hydrosols (page 46)

INGREDIENTS

1 quart (1 liter) warm water (100° F)

2 cups (500 ml) mint tea

2 cups (500 ml) chamomile tea

2 cups (500 ml) rosemary infusion

1 tablespoon sea salt

1 teaspoon grated ginger

½ teaspoon (2.5 ml) tea tree oil

1 tablespoon grape seed oil

Note: You can substitute olive oil for grape seed oil, depending on availability.

INSTRUCTIONS

1. Pour all ingredients (except the grape seed oil) into a wide foot spa or basin.

2. Make sure the water temperature is warm and pleasant. Soak your feet for 30 minutes.

3. Dry them with a towel and use a pumice stone to soften the skin and remove dead skin cells. Finish by massaging the feet with the grape seed oil.

Foot Odor Neutralizing Formula

Have you ever thought of soaking your beauty brushes in white vinegar to clean and sanitize them? Well, this foot odor–killing recipe will make you appreciate the power of white vinegar. Mint contains menthol, which is refreshing and complements the odor-neutralizing properties of the lavender essential oil.

INGREDIENTS

2 quarts (2 liters) hot water (100° F)

2 cups (500 ml) mint tea

1 cup white vinegar

2 tablespoons sea salt

½ teaspoon (2.5 ml) lavender essential oil

INSTRUCTIONS

1. Pour the water into a basin. Add the remaining ingredients, making sure to dissolve the salt.

2. Soak your feet, sit back, and relax for 10 minutes. Rinse your feet with plain water and pat them dry with a towel. Finish with a foot balm.

3. For longer-lasting results, repeat this foot bath on a weekly basis.

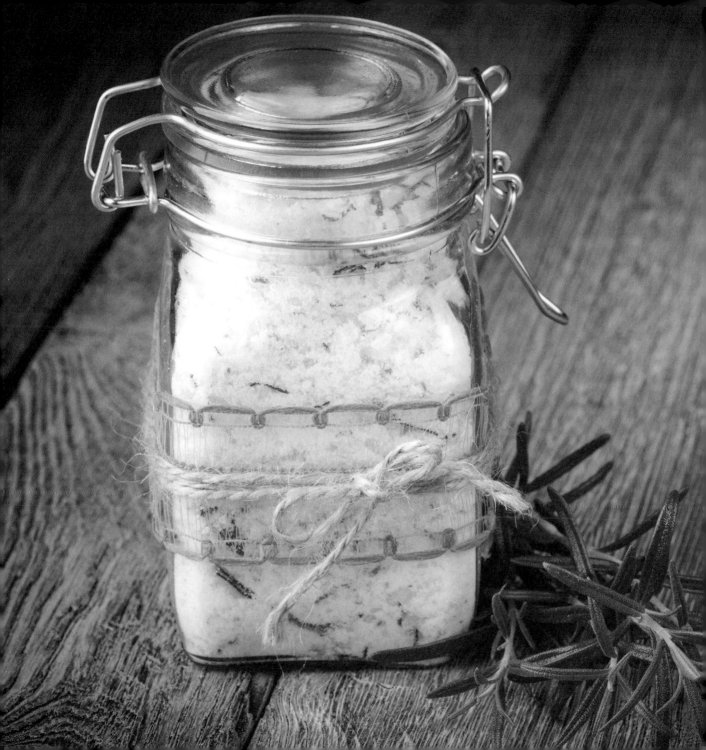

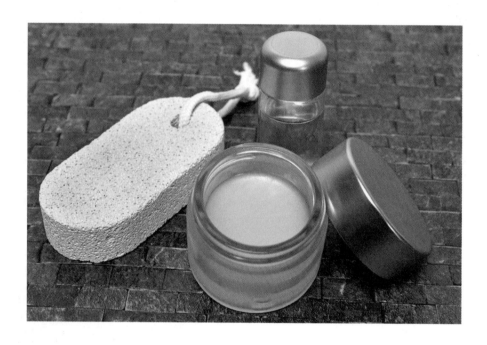

Cracked Heels Balm

The skin that covers the heels is thick and presents a strong barrier to moisturizers and creams. Regular foot care, including the use of a pumice stone, and a powerful balm are important to maintain soft heels.

INGREDIENTS

- 1 ounce (30 ml) grated beeswax (or pellets)
- 1 ounce (30 ml) shea butter
- 3 ounces (100 ml) almond oil
- 2 ounces (60 ml) olive oil
- ½ teaspoon lavender essential oil

INSTRUCTIONS

1. In a double boiler, melt the beeswax and shea butter.

2. In another double boiler, heat the almond and olive oils, bringing both mixtures to a similar temperature (100–120°F). Measure this using a candy thermometer. Turn off the heat under the oils and slowly pour them into the beeswax mixture, whisking constantly.

3. Turn off the heat under the beeswax, add the lavender essential oil, and continue whisking.

4. Transfer the mixture to a tin box or glass jar, pouring slowly to release any trapped air. Wait for the balm to reach room temperature before sealing the lid. Set aside to solidify.

5. Apply a quarter-size amount of balm to each foot and rub it all over your feet, focusing on the heel area. Rub a small amount of balm on your heels for a minute or two to improve its penetration through the skin. Wear spa socks to help keep the feet soft and moisturized.

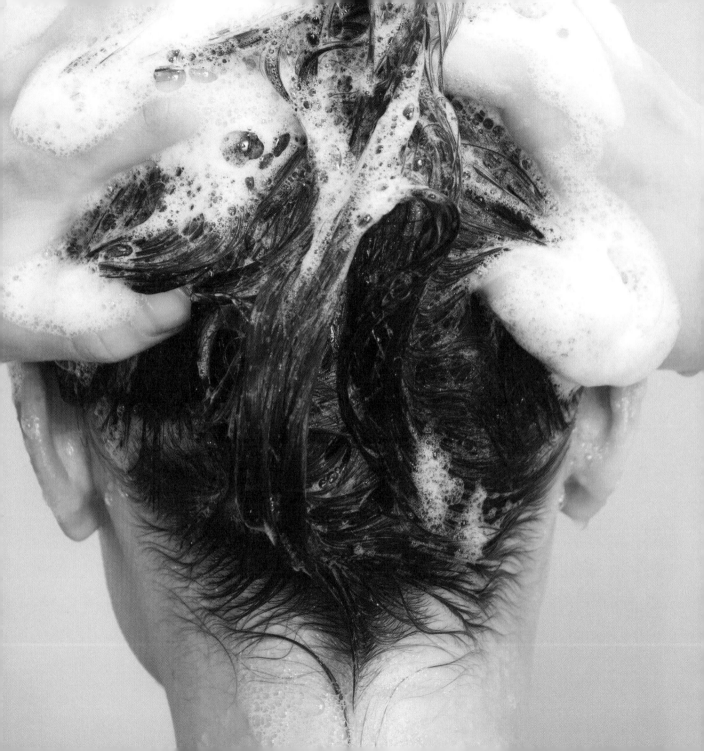

CHAPTER 15

Hair Care

Multiple formulas are offered in this chapter to nourish your hair and scalp, and many of them are customized to meet the needs of specific hair types, in natural ways that maintain hair strength, bounce, and shine.

Subtle Bubble Shampoo

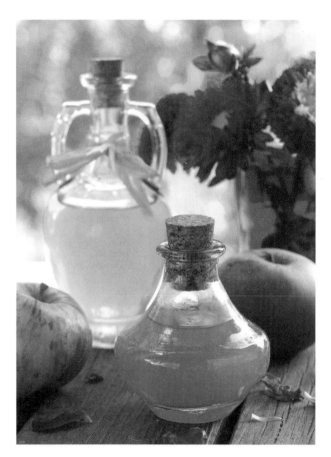

This formula will transform concentrated liquid soap into a smooth and balanced hair shampoo. The argan oil restores shine and luster to dull hair.

See How to Make Your Own Infusions, Decoctions, and Hydrosols (page 46)

INGREDIENTS

½ cup rosemary infusion (cooled)
1 teaspoon apple cider vinegar, for pH adjustment
2 ounces (60 ml) liquid castile soap
1 teaspoon argan oil

INSTRUCTIONS

1. Mix the rosemary infusion and the vinegar. Then pour it into the soap base, in a thin stream, whisking very gently to prevent foaming. Blend in the argan oil, slowly, still whisking until all ingredients are well blended.

2. Use as a regular shampoo.

Blond Hair Shampoo

This shampoo is good for all hair types, but especially blond hair, because the chamomile will enhance its natural color. Glycerin will soften the hair and keep it moisturized.

INGREDIENTS

1 cup freshly made chamomile tea

1 teaspoon vegetable-derived glycerin

1 teaspoon white vinegar

1 ounce (30 ml) vegetable soap flakes (you can use a cheese grater to grate a bar of soap)

INSTRUCTIONS

1. Mix all the ingredients except the soap.

2. While the tea mixture is still warm, sprinkle the soap flakes on the surface and mix well. Then transfer the final mixture to a bottle.

3. Shake well prior to shampooing. Rinse with water after using, as with all shampoos.

Quick Hair Rinse

This formula is suitable for oily hair, because the astringency of the green tea will help tame sebum secretion. It is a watery mixture of rosemary hydrosol, white vinegar, and green tea and will give your hair vitality and shine. Vinegar adjusts the pH of the preparation.

See How to Make Your Own Infusions, Decoctions, and Hydrosols (page 46)

INGREDIENTS

3 ounces (100 ml) green tea infusion

3 ounces (100 ml) rosemary infusion

1 teaspoon white vinegar

INSTRUCTIONS

1. Mix all the above ingredients and transfer the mixture to a spray bottle.

2. Use as a hair rinse after shampooing. Spray liberally on your hair, leave on for a couple of minutes, and then rinse with plain water.

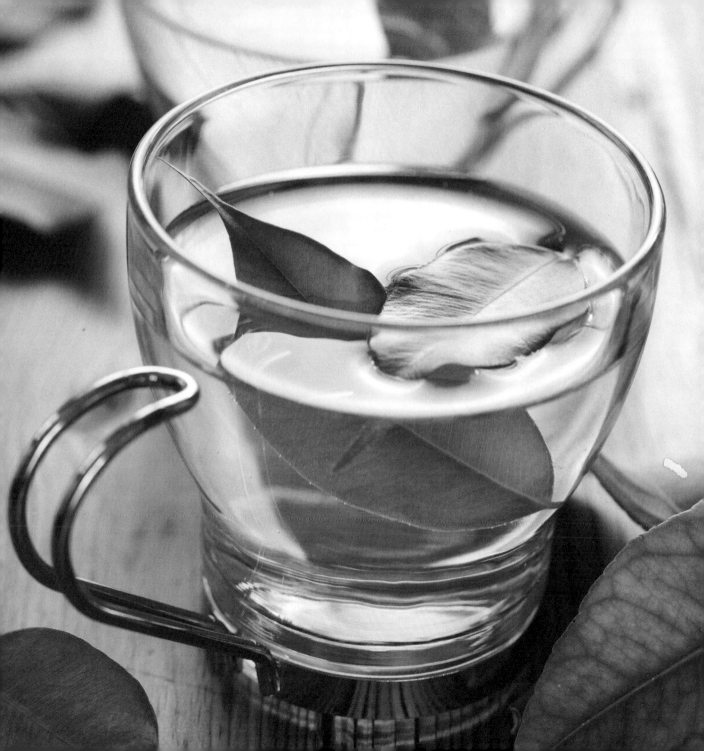

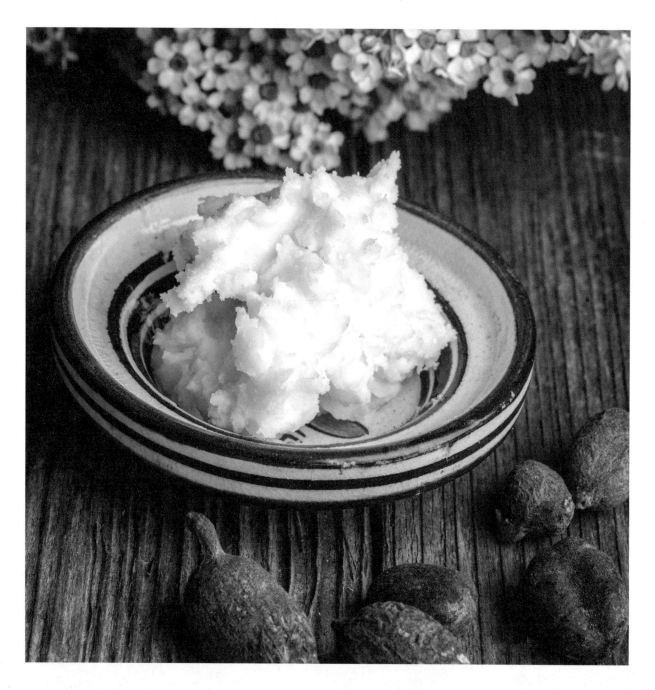

Soft and Silky Conditioner

This extremely softening hair conditioner works as a leave-in cream and requires no rinsing. It controls frizz and helps achieve defined curls.

INGREDIENTS

2 ounces (60 ml) shea butter

1 teaspoon emulsifier (such as glyceryl stearate)

1 ounce (30 ml) rosemary hydrosol

INSTRUCTIONS

1. Use a double boiler to soften the shea butter over low heat. When the butter becomes liquid, add the emulsifier. Use another double boiler to heat the rosemary hydrosol. Monitor the temperature using a candy thermometer. When both solutions reach a temperature of 175° F, turn off the heat under both pans, and pour the hydrosol into the shea butter mixture slowly, steadily, and in a thin stream, whisking vigorously the whole time. Continue whisking until the mixture reaches room temperature; then transfer it to a small jar.

2. After showering, while your hair is still wet, rub a dab of this conditioner on your fingers and run them through your hair. Avoid using too much if you want to preserve some hair volume. Comb and style as usual.

Color-Treated Hair Oil

This *bain d'huile* will soften colored hair and give it back its shine and manageability. Make this oily hair mask every couple of months, mainly after aggressive hair treatment or if you have dry brittle hair. Moroccan argan oil and rosemary oil are excellent hair ingredients; make sure you include them in this formula to give luster, bounce, and strength to your hair.

INGREDIENTS

    1 ounce (30 ml) almond oil
    1 ounce (30 ml) jojoba oil
    1 teaspoon argan oil
    10 drops (0.5 ml) rosemary essential oil

INSTRUCTIONS

1. Mix all of the above ingredients and transfer the mixture to an amber bottle.

2. To use, apply a small amount to wet hair during your shower. Run your fingers through your hair to coat the hair with oil and massage it into your scalp for best absorption.

3. Put on a plastic shower cap and wait for 20–30 minutes before shampooing your hair twice.

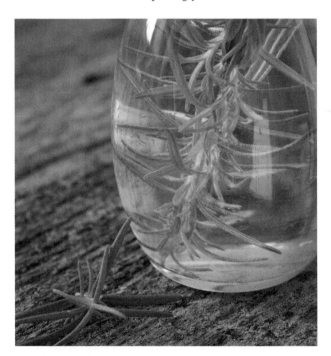

Leave-In Anti-Frizz Hair Spray

This formula relies on the humectant properties of glycerin, which draws moisture and works as a silky coat for frizzy hair. Rose water hydrosol is a soft and fragrant ingredient that suits most hair types.

INGREDIENTS

2 ounces (60 ml) distilled or purified water

2 ounces (60 ml) rose water

1 tablespoon vegetable-derived glycerin

10 drops (0.5 ml) geranium or lavender essential oil (optional)

INSTRUCTIONS

1. Whisk all ingredients together until well blended and transfer the mixture to a spray bottle.

2. Prior to spraying on wet or dry hair, shake vigorously. Style as usual.

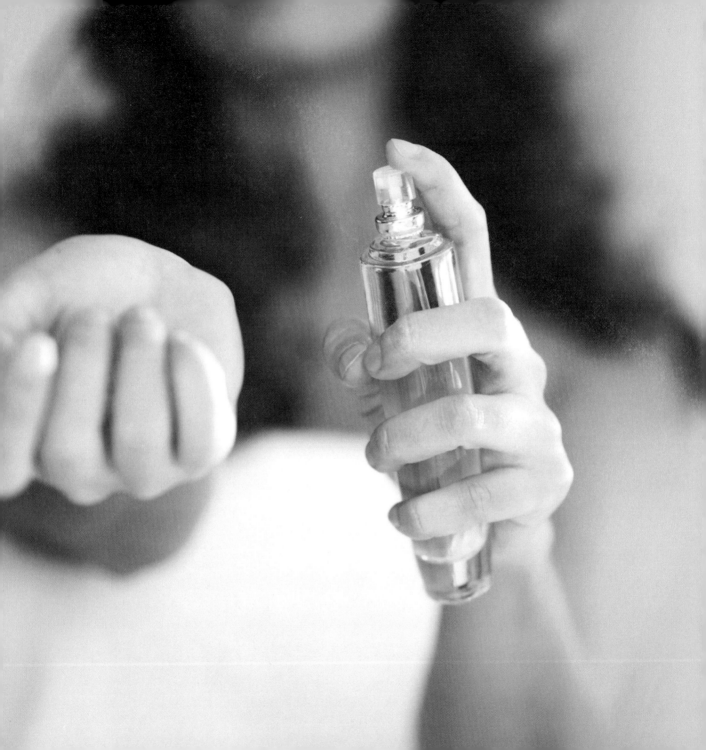

CHAPTER 16

Perfumes and Scented Sprays

Making your own perfume is an art. The basic ingredients are always the same and preparation is easy, as long as you know how to combine the essential oils to reach your preferred scent.

As a rule of thumb, mainly for beginners, start with two or three essential oils. Once you have mastered this art, and feel more confident, you can juggle more essential oils of different categories to give depth to your eau de toilette.

A "well-structured" perfume has deep notes (also referred to as bottom or base notes), complemented by middle (or heart) notes, and top notes.

Vanilla, musk, patchouli, and frankincense are examples of essential oils that can provide a solid base for your perfume. Deep notes should make up about 50 percent of your blend. Those aromas will linger for the whole day. Middle notes will actually bond the deep notes and top notes together. They will transport you through the perfume journey. A good proportion for heart notes is 30 percent. You can throw into your blend some magnolia, gardenia,

rose, jasmine, rosemary, or ylang-ylang for a full-bodied scent. Finish with 20 percent of top notes. Those are the notes that will overwhelm your senses at first and then fade to bring in the deeper notes. Think of lighter fragrances for your top notes, floral or citrus, fresh and light, such as tangerine, lime, bergamot, cherry, apple, peach, and so forth.

You could start with a sampler kit and play with its essential oils until you are ready to invest in a bigger collection.

Try a blend of geranium, gardenia, jasmine, and rose essential oils for a spring flowery scent. Alternatively, try a blend of lemon, lemon balm, citronella, bergamot, and orange blossom essential oils for a citrusy, uplifting fragrance. If you like deeper notes, then cedar wood, sandalwood, and patchouli essential oils might be your choice. For a warm, yummy scent, incorporate vanilla, cinnamon, nutmeg, and clove essential oils.

Because essential oils are extremely concentrated (100 percent pure), make sure you work in a properly ventilated area. Do not inhale undiluted essential oils, and always read about the benefits and hazards of your essential oils before you start manipulating them. It is not advisable to put essential oils directly on the skin unless they are first diluted with a carrier oil to avoid sensitization.

Once you have created one or more scents that satisfy your senses, you will need to dilute them into an actual perfume. Because rubbing alcohol evaporates, it is a great carrier for a scent. Blend it with water for a more fragrant result. Vodka is also a good substitute for rubbing alcohol; even the cheapest vodka is food grade, which makes it superior to commercial rubbing alcohol and less polluted with unwanted chemicals. You can also make an alcohol-free perfume, using instead an ingredient such as propanediol or cyclomethicone, or simply a carrier oil of your choice, such as jojoba, for a natural oil perfume.

Your Own Oil Perfume

Once you have created a scent that speaks to your senses, transforming it into a perfume is a breeze. Oil perfumes are easy to make and can be more concentrated than volatile fragrances.

INGREDIENTS

3 tablespoons (50 ml) jojoba oil
20 drops (1 ml) your own essential oils blend

INSTRUCTIONS

1. Pour the jojoba oil into a small roll-on container, or a dropper bottle. Add your essential oils, fasten the lid, and shake well. Let the oils fuse for a day or two.

2. Place a couple of drops of your perfume on warm body spots, such as behind the ears and on the inside of the wrists.

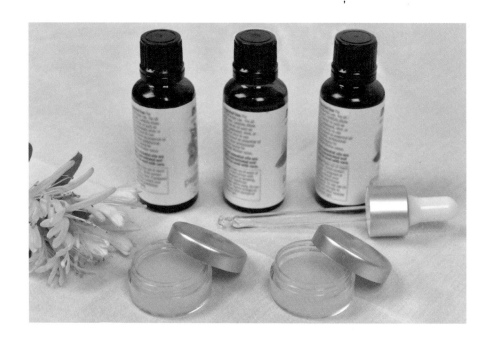

Solid Perfume

Perfumed balms are easy to make and store well. Three main ingredients are needed: a solid base such as beeswax or shea butter; a liquid oil that will soften the solid phase, such as almond oil, olive oil, or jojoba oil; and a scent made by mixing a few of your favorite essential oils.

INGREDIENTS

3 ounces (100 ml) shea butter

1 ounce (30 ml) almond oil

½ teaspoon tangerine essential oil

½ teaspoon grapefruit essential oil

20 drops (1 ml) peppermint essential oil

INSTRUCTIONS

1. In a double boiler, melt the shea butter, and then add the almond oil. Mix quickly with a whisk, turn off the heat, and continue whisking as you add the essential oils.

2. Transfer the mixture to a tin box and allow it to cool before fastening the lid.

3. Use as a solid perfume by rubbing little amounts on warm body spots such as behind the ears and inside the wrists.

Custom Eau de Toilette

It is very easy to make your own eau de toilette at a fraction of the cost and with fully known ingredients and all-natural fragrances.

INGREDIENTS

2 ounces (60 ml) distilled water

1 ounce (30 ml) rubbing alcohol

½ teaspoon your own essential oils blend

INSTRUCTIONS

1. Create your own essential oils using solid ingredients such as cinnamon sticks, nutmeg, cloves, or lemon rind or zest, drop them into a glass jar, cover with rubbing alcohol, seal the lid, and leave for a week, away from sunlight and in a cool place. Shake frequently to help the oils transfer into the alcohol. Then filter through a cheesecloth and transfer to an amber bottle.

2. If you are using a blend of essential oils, allow the scents to "fuse" for a couple of days before adding them to your mixture.

3. Mix the water and essential oils, shake well, and store in a dark-colored glass perfume bottle.

4. Use this mixture as you would any other eau de toilette. Do not spray on the face or on irritated skin.

Fresh Scent Body Spray

The perspiration caused by summer heat can be embarrassing, and a handy body spray can be a great relief. This recipe combines the fresh, clean smell of citrusy ingredients with the astringent effects of witch hazel and the antiseptic properties of green tea. Rubbing alcohol or vodka will help reduce the bacterial load on the skin surface and counteract body odor.

INGREDIENTS

½ cup rubbing alcohol or vodka

2 ounces (60 ml) witch hazel

2 ounces (60 ml) green tea

20 drops (1 ml) grapefruit essential oil

20 drops (1 ml) tangerine essential oil

Note: You can substitute lavender essential oil for the citrusy essential oils in this recipe for a more gender-neutral scent.

INSTRUCTIONS

1. Mix all the above ingredients and transfer the mixture to a spray bottle.

2. Allow the ingredients to "fuse" for a couple of days before using.

3. Use this spray every day, if you like, especially on hot days when you've been perspiring. Always shake the bottle before spraying.

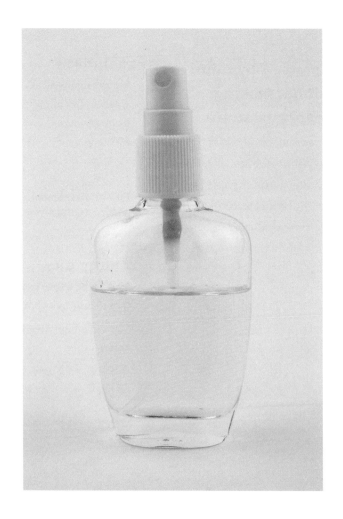

Odor-Neutralizing Spray

Body odor develops as the body releases accumulated toxins through sweat and sebum secretions. Since the skin folds are poorly ventilated, skin flora (bacteria normally present on the skin surface) tends to proliferate within those folds, where moisture and sweat are optimal.

Baking soda is a strong odor-neutralizing agent. It has multiple domestic uses such as eliminating odors, as a laundry detergent ingredient, and, of course, in baking. It also has cosmetic applications, including deodorants for odor control. The addition of two antiseptic essential oils will allow for the disinfecting effect of rubbing alcohol and limit bacterial proliferation. This synergistic effect is maximized by the addition of an astringent agent that will reduce the size of skin pores and limit the secretion of sebum. The addition of glycerin will counteract the drying effect of the rubbing alcohol.

INGREDIENTS

2 ounces (60 ml) witch hazel
2 ounces (60 ml) green tea
2 ounces (60 ml) rubbing alcohol
1 teaspoon vegetable-derived glycerin
10 drops (0.5 ml) tea tree essential oil
10 drops (0.5 ml) thyme essential oil
1 tablespoon baking soda

INSTRUCTIONS

1. Pour all the liquid ingredients into a spray bottle. Slowly add the baking soda. Shake the bottle gently to dissolve and mix all the ingredients.

2. Shake the bottle vigorously before each use. Spray one to two times under the arms and allow the moisture to dry before dressing.

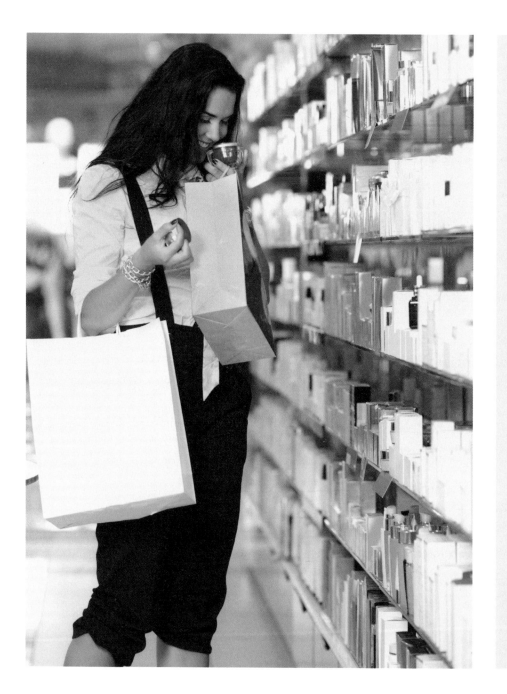

3

Buying Commercial Skin Care Products

Choosing to buy commercial products doesn't have to compromise your love for natural ingredients; especially with the boom in "natural" and "organic" products. Recognizing these products on store shelves, or online, among a multitude of substandard intruders, can be a real challenge. The information presented in the next three chapters will serve as a guide, helping you make wiser choices by knowing what to avoid and what to look for, as well as how to differentiate truly natural products from wannabes and identify authentic certified claims.

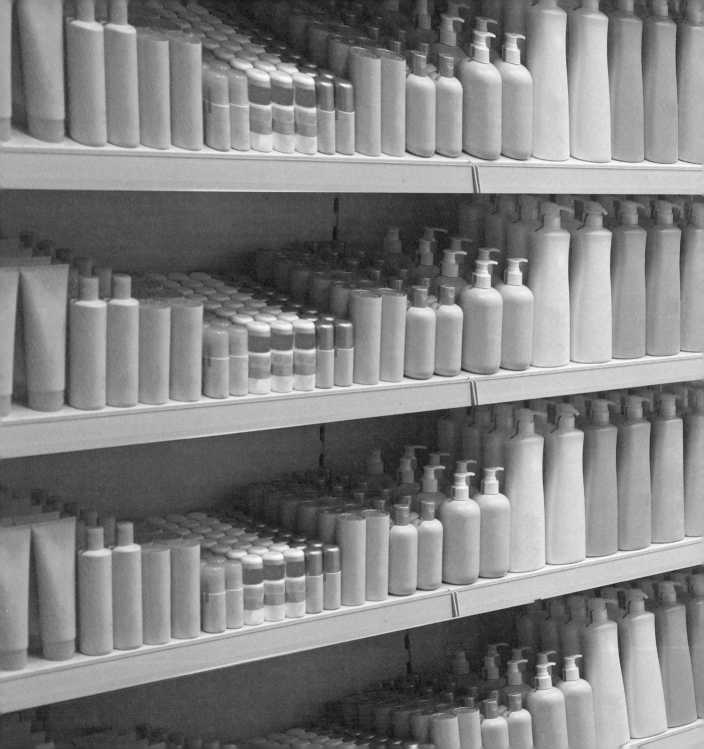

CHAPTER 17

Debated Ingredients

A major driver behind the will to buy more natural products is the awareness that some ingredients and chemicals included in commercial products could pose health hazards. With weak regulations, and the FDA's limited role, manufacturers enjoy a large amount of freedom in formulating their cosmetics.

The Federal Food, Drug, and Cosmetic Act (FD&C) defines cosmetics by their intended use, as "articles intended to be rubbed, poured, sprinkled, or sprayed on, introduced into, or otherwise applied to the human body . . . for cleansing, beautifying, promoting attractiveness, or altering the appearance." With the exception of authorized colors and sunscreens (for which proof of SPF level is required), the vast majority of cosmetics remain poorly regulated. The FDA has not been able to impose regulations pertaining to cosmetics the way it has for pharmaceuticals, mainly because the cosmetics lobby has succeeded in protecting the industry's interests from such constraints. Lack of regulation and continued use of ingredients banned in other parts of the world, such as the European Union, Japan, and Sweden, incited multiple organizations, such as the Environmental Working Group, to interact with legislators in an attempt to create some order.

The resulting Safe Cosmetics Act (introduced in June 2011) aimed at avoiding harmful ingredients, making personal care products safer for both workers and consumers, and requiring full disclosure of ingredients. The act also encouraged ingredient safety data-sharing, and the development of alternatives to animal testing.

With increasing reports on the poor safety profiles of certain ingredients and the failure of some studies to demonstrate their inoffensiveness, a lot of noise has been made to warn consumers, mainly women, about the potential hazards of those ingredients. Even though there are numerous data gaps, and often not enough solid research to draw conclusive results, many ingredients have been under fire for a while and for various reasons. Most of those ingredients are listed and discussed in the following paragraphs.

Aluminum

Aluminum is a ubiquitous metal that is widely used in cookware, antacids, and antiperspirants. Even though it seems to be less toxic than other heavy metals, there are concerns related to chronic aluminum toxicity. Because some studies have shown higher deposits of aluminum in the brain plaque of people with Alzheimer's disease, it is thought to be linked to Alzheimer's. Evidence is still inconclusive, however, as to whether the deposit is a cause or a consequence of the condition. Aluminum is also a metalloestrogen, which means that it is a metal that has some estrogenic activity; that is why there are concerns arising from its use in antiperspirants.

Avobenzone

Avobenzone is an oil-soluble dibenzoylmethane derivative that belongs to the class of chemical sunscreens. While mineral sunscreens (zinc oxide, titanium dioxide) reflect UV light, chemical sunscreens absorb it. Avobenzone is effective in absorbing UVAs, but it is photosensitive; sun exposure promotes its disintegration, which compromises its efficacy. One single hour of sun exposure can lead to the loss of more than a third of the avobenzone initially present. Manufacturers have tried to counteract this by adding photo-stabilizers, such as octocrylene, to the formulation. The much higher stability of mineral sunscreens, however, as well as their limited absorption through the skin, has led to their increased popularity versus chemical sunscreens such as avobenzone.

Benzalkonium Chloride

This is a commonly used, potent antimicrobial, with applications ranging from eye drop preservative to household cleaners. It is used in various hand sanitizers, disinfecting wipes, pharmaceutical antiseptics, mouthwash, among other products.

The typical concentration in eye drops ranges from 0.002 to 0.01 percent. Studies suggest that concentrations of 0.02 percent or more can denature corneal protein and inflict irreversible damage on the eyes. Concentrations within the usage range may lead to corneal punctures.

Benzalkonium chloride is also a skin-sensitizing agent. Concentrations of 10 percent or more are capable of producing a strong irritation to the skin and mucous membranes; it is potentially lethal when taken internally. Benzalkonium chloride has been used for decades to disinfect cuts and wounds because it is less painful than rubbing alcohol when applied.

Benzoic Acid and Sodium Benzoate

Sodium benzoate is obtained by neutralizing benzoic acid with sodium hydroxide or sodium bicarbonate. Even though benzoic acid is a more effective preservative, sodium benzoate is more commonly used because it has better water solubility. Sodium benzoate (also called E211) is used as a bacteriostatic and fungistatic in acidic foods and beverages, cosmetics, and pharmaceutical preparations. The FDA requires a maximum concentration of 0.1 percent. The International Program on Chemical Safety found no adverse effects of daily doses ranging from 647 to 825mg/kg of body weight.

Sodium benzoate reacts with ascorbic acid (vitamin C, or E300) and yields benzene, which is a known carcinogen. Soft drinks have very low concentrations of sodium benzoate, and some companies are phasing it out. Poor storage conditions—in heat and light, for example—increase the speed at which benzene is formed.

BHT and BHA

BHT (butylated hydroxytoluene, also known as E321) is used as a food additive to maintain freshness. It is also commonly used in cosmetics and pharmaceutical preparations. It is thought to be linked to hyperactivity disorder, with conflicting data in regards to its carcinogenicity. Some food brands have chosen to exclude it from their ingredients; others have chosen to replace it with BHA.

BHA (butylated hydroxyanisole, or E320) is also a food additive, with applications similar to those of BHT. Data behind BHA is controversial and limited. The state of California, however, has listed BHA as a known carcinogen.

Borax

Borax (E285) is a naturally occurring element that is widely used in an array of industrial and chemical applications. It is a fire retardant, buffering agent, laundry booster, ant bait, preservative, and more. It is banned for use as a food additive in the United States but is still used in some other countries. Borax is among the ingredients of many natural cosmetics sold on the U.S. market. The European Union has classified it as "toxic for reproduction" and requires a printed warning on all borax-containing preparations.

Colors

FD&C colors are synthetic colorings that have been approved by the FDA for use in foods, beverages, cosmetics, and drugs. Each of the nine approved synthetic dyes has a specific FD&C number. Synthetic food colorings are preferred by some manufacturers over naturally derived colors because they are cheaper and do not affect flavor.

The safety of synthetic dyes has been evaluated by many national and international groups, with various conclusions and opinions. The main concern is their link to an increased prevalence of ADD (attention deficit disorder) and ADHD (attention deficit and hyperactivity disorder). Even though studies have not been able to demonstrate a causal link, some studies have shown better academic performance in non-ADD groups when such food additives were eliminated.

There are many highly purified, naturally derived colorants that can be incorporated into foods and personal care products. Naturally derived colors include annatto, beet, caramel, chlorophyllin, turmeric, and beta-carotene, among others. There may be carryover ingredients (mainly extraction solvents) in the final color, but the percentage is usually so low that it is not obligatory to mention it on the label.

Coal Tar

Coal tar is a thick black liquid, a by-product of the coal industry. It is a blend of hundreds of different organic compounds, not all of which have been identified. It is considered an OTC (over the counter) pharmaceutical drug and is used in lotions and shampoos to treat dandruff, psoriasis, and head lice. Coal tar is a known carcinogen, especially in preparations in which it exceeds 5 percent concentration.

Dihydroxyacetone

Dihydroxyacetone (DHA) is the most widely used ingredient in sunless tanners. It reacts with the amino acids of epidermal skin cells to produce a melanin-like color. Most products contain 3–5 percent DHA, although some professional products may contain up to 15 percent.

Even though the FDA has approved DHA for topical use, the agency has issued a warning to avoid accidental swallowing or inhaling it when it's applied as a mist in sun booths. Some reports have demonstrated an increase in free radicals after application, as well as cell-damaging effects. There is also some decrease in vitamin D production through the skin.

Hydroquinone

This skin-lightening ingredient is banned in Europe and many other regions of the world. It is still included in many OTC preparations in the United States, however, even though the FDA has declared that it cannot be ruled out as a potential human carcinogen. It is also a strong skin sensitizer poorly tolerated by sensitive skin.

Formaldehyde and formaldehyde-releasing agents

Formaldehyde (chemically called methanal) is a gaseous aldehyde that is colorless and has a pungent smell. Commercial solutions of formaldehyde in water are called formaline and are used to preserve animal tissues. Formaldehyde is a fixative and an embalming agent. It is used in woodwork and many other products. It is also widely used in the medical field as a biocide (except where banned, as in the European Union). Other related compounds, such as imidazolidinyl urea, diazolidinyl urea, and DMDM hydantoin are capable or releasing formaldehyde. The U.S. national toxicology program considers formaldehyde to be a known human carcinogen. It is also a respiratory irritant and a skin-sensitizing agent, which might cause dermatitis. It is present in many personal care products, such as keratin hair treatments, whose use is considered an occupational hazard by some hair care professionals.

Mineral Oil

Also known as white oil, liquid paraffin, and liquid petroleum, mineral oil is a by-product of crude oil distillation. It is produced in large quantities and has a relatively low price. White petroleum is a solid form of mineral oil and is also known as petroleum jelly. Unrefined and poorly refined mineral oils are classified as carcinogenic to humans by the World Health Organization. Theoretically, the risk decreases as purity increases. Refined oils are widely used in cosmetics, in which they act as moisturizers and emollients. Mineral oil is also used as a makeup remover because of its solvent properties.

Monoethanolamine, Diethanolamine, and Triethanolamine

Monoethanolamine (MEA or EDA) is a corrosive and toxic liquid. It is a weak base used as a buffering agent in some pharmaceutical emulsions. Excessive, prolonged, or widespread exposure through the skin may result in kidney or liver damage.

Diethanolamine (DEA or DEOA) is used in the production of diethanolamides such as cocamide DEA, lauramide DEA, oleamide DEA, myristamide DEA, and DEA cetyl phosphate, which are widely used in cosmetics and shampoos to improve the creamy texture and the foaming capacity. Skin irritation and sensitization are the primary concerns arising from DEA-containing products.

Triethanolamine (TEA or TEOA) is a stronger base used as a buffering agent in many cosmetics to adjust the final pH of the product. It is also a surfactant and an emulsifier. When added to facial cleansers, for example, it improves makeup removal. It is also added to many other products, such as laundry detergents, liquid cleaners, polishes, and others. Because it may convert to nitrosamines, which are known carcinogens, its use has raised concerns. It is also a strong allergen.

Musk

Musk is a naturally occurring, highly fragrant substance that has long been used in perfumery. Natural sources are mainly animal, such as the musk deer (from musk-secreting glands), and botanical (plants, flowers, or seeds). However, because of the scarcity of these natural resources and the increasing demand, synthetic musk, also called white musk, has been developed and has replaced natural musk almost totally. Most kinds of synthetic musk (such as musk-xylene) are suspected carcinogens, and there are efforts to replace them with less harmful types.

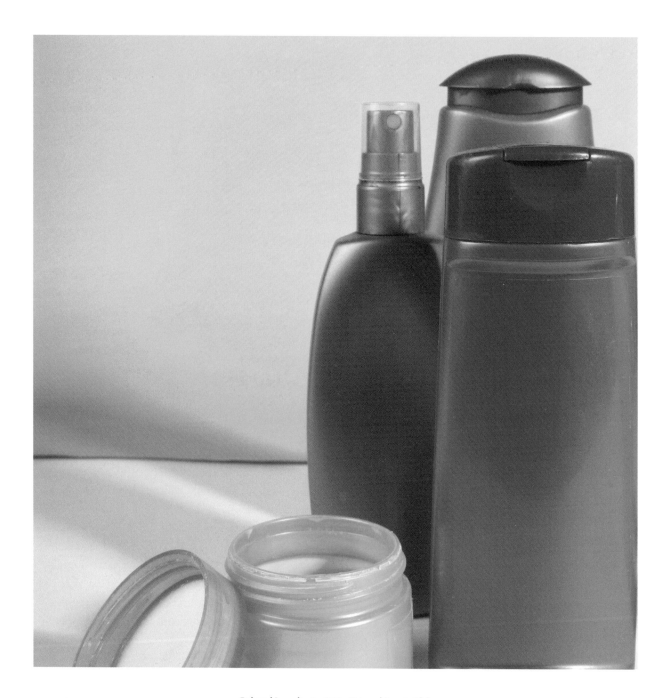

Nanoparticles in Sunscreens

New technologies have allowed a reduction of the size of particles in sunscreens to micron and nano levels. These practices create much smaller sized particles with multiple pharmaceutical and industrial applications. Nanoparticle diameter ranges from 1 to 100 nanometers. Pharmaceutical formulations using nanoparticles capable of penetrating biological membranes promise enhanced delivery of the active ingredient and superior targeting.

In cosmetics, the most famous nanoparticle is zinc oxide. Zinc oxide is a naturally occurring element that is widely used in mineral sunscreens, mineral makeup, and diaper rash creams. Its initial-size molecule is not absorbed into the skin and is capable of reflecting UVAs and UVBs from the skin surface. However, reducing the size of the zinc oxide molecule tremendously increases the surface versus volume, rendering those particles unstable and highly reactive. Their effects at the cellular level have raised safety concerns, especially as some studies have established their mutagenicity and cytotoxicity. The depth of skin penetration remains poorly established.

While the FDA is still investigating the safety of nanoparticles in cosmetics, many manufacturers have voluntarily chosen to withhold them from their formulas. Labeling regulations do not require specifying whether zinc oxide is micronized, nano, or regular size, and consumers are left to research that information.

PABA

Para-aminobenzoic acid (PABA) is a chemical ingredient used mainly in sunscreens and included in numerous oral supplements. The FDA has not determined a recommended daily intake for PABA, and the health benefits of oral supplementation remain vague. As for its use in sunscreens, it is losing its popularity as a chemical UVA and UVB filter because of the high incidence of allergic reactions among consumers. Also, the emergence of negative reports on PABA's mutagenicity has led to its replacement by other chemical and mineral filters.

Parabens

Parabens are esters of parahydroxybenzoic acid. Paraben-based preservatives include methylparaben (E218), ethylparaben (E214), propylparaben (E216), and butylparaben. Germaben, Germaben II, Phenonip, and other types, such as Germall and LiquaPar Oil, are alternative names for paraben-based preservatives. Parabens have slight estrogenic activity, which means that they can weakly mimic the natural female hormone estrogen. This is why they are said to be endocrine disruptors and have been found in breast cancer tissue. Even though parabens do have estrogenic activity, in vivo (in humans) activity remains weak compared to the activity of estrogen itself.

Phenoxyethanol

Phenoxyethanol is a preservative used in a great number of skin care and makeup products. It is also used in a number of biological drugs and pharmaceutical preparations.

It can cause skin allergies and might depress the central nervous system; it may lead to vomiting and diarrhea (in high concentrations). It is considered safe by many manufacturers, however, and is approved for all ages.

Phthalates

Phthalates are esters of phthalic acid with short- or long-chain radicals. They are mainly used as plasticizers in applications from pharmaceutical pills and medical supplies to toys, paints, nail polish, perfumes, shower curtains, packaging materials, and more. Diethyl and dibutyl phthalates are the main two phthalates present in personal care products.

While some European countries are banning the use of phthalates, they remain ubiquitous and even though they do not accumulate in nature, they are common pollutants of homes, especially in urban and suburban areas. They evaporate and are easily released into the immediate environment. They can be inhaled, ingested with food, and absorbed through the skin. Carcinogenicity, birth defects, endocrine disruption, asthma, and behavioral changes are among the health concerns raised by phthalates.

Synthetic Fragrances

Fragrance is often added to products to mask an unpleasant odor or to impart a pleasant smell.

Sometimes it is added to a gas such as propane to make potential leaks noticeable.

The chemical name of a synthetic fragrance (or blend of fragrances) does not have to be mentioned on the ingredients label of a product, which is a source of concern for some consumers. There are various chemical categories of fragrances, such as terpenes, aldehydes, esters, amines, alcohols, ketones, and lactones.

Fragrance components are both inhaled and absorbed through the skin, and many are highly sensitizing, which means that they are capable of triggering allergies and dermatitis. Many fragrance chemicals are also endocrine disruptors (affecting mainly estrogen and thyroid hormones), bio-accumulating substances (substances that accumulate in the human body, especially in fat tissues), and simply unevaluated components that are often not listed on labels.

The perfume industry relies on thousands of chemicals, sometimes natural but mostly synthetic, to compound various scents. Many ingredients are petroleum-derived. The Research Institute for Fragrance Materials does assess the safety of many chemicals used in the fragrance industry, but many components remain unstudied.

People with asthma or migraines might be less tolerant of specific scents. Essential oils, which are much more expensive than fragrances, are still often preferred in natural skin care because of their better tolerability profile and natural origins.

Talcum Powder

Talcum powder (magnesium silicate) is a naturally occurring whitish substance with a wide array of applications. In cosmetics, it serves as a lubricant and an astringent powder. Long used for diaper rash, talcum powder became less popular after a link to ovarian and lung cancer was suspected. There have also been toxicity reports due to impurities in talcum powder.

Titanium Dioxide

Titanium dioxide is a naturally occurring white pigment used in multiple industrial, pharmaceutical, and cosmetic applications. It is also an approved food additive. Titanium dioxide is a reactive pigment that generates damaging free radicals. It is coated with silica or alumina to prevent the acceleration of a photoreaction. A number of commercially available mineral-based sunscreens offer titanium-free option to consumers.

Triclosan

This ingredient was initially developed as a surgical scrubbing agent and has gained popularity as the active ingredient in many disinfecting products such as soaps, hand sanitizers, mouthwashes, toothpastes, and disinfecting wipes.

Some studies have shown that triclosan might compromise the immune system, cause allergies, and make humans more susceptible to the hazardous effects of BPA (bisphenol A, commonly present in plastics and the lining of food cans). Other studies have shown that it affects muscles in other animal species, and there may be similar concerns for humans. The FDA is reviewing the safety of triclosan.

Note that washing your hands for 20–30 seconds with soap and water or using a hand sanitizer with 60 percent or more alcohol content is an effective and reliable way to kill most common germs.

Other Ingredients

Many other ingredients—propylene glycol, polyethylene glycol (PEG), isopropyl alcohol (rubbing alcohol), silicones, and others—have been criticized for various reasons. Most of those products have various pharmaceutical and medical applications. It is very important, however, for such ingredients to be produced according to solid GMP (good manufacturing practice) standards and yield highly purified products quasi-free from contaminants that might compromise the quality of the product.

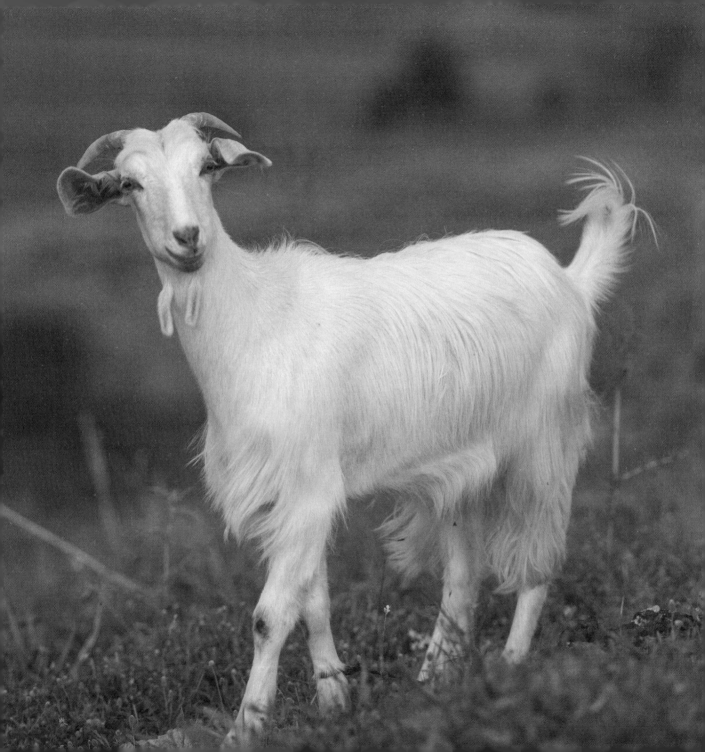

CHAPTER 18

Animal-Derived Ingredients

Another category of ingredients poorly welcomed among natural beauty lovers is animal-derived ingredients, which are universally present in cosmetics, with applications ranging from mere emulsifiers to dermal fillers. Many consumers prefer to exclude animal by-products from their skin care products, mostly because of veganism or because of heavy processing and possible contamination of such ingredients. Usually, products that are free of animal by-products say "vegan friendly" on the packaging. Manufacturers should also specify the source of an ingredient if it could be either animal or non-animal derived.

The animal by-products listed in the following paragraphs are among the most commonly used in the cosmetics industry:

Albumin

Albumin is a major blood plasma protein, also present in egg whites. Mostly bovine-sourced, it is used in cosmetics for its wrinkle-smoothing effect.

Carmine

Also known as cochineal, crimson lake, or E120, this deep red pigment, used in food and makeup, is derived from carminic acid obtained from the scales of insects.

Collagen and Gelatin

Collagen is a protein that makes up the majority of connective tissues in animals. It is widely used in cosmetic surgeries as a dermal filler and in many other medical applications. Gelatin is used in cosmetics as a non-gelling, thickening or film-forming agent. It is often listed as hydrolyzed collagen. Collagen can also be marine sourced, from fish. It is often sold as a powder and included in anti-aging creams.

Elastin

As its name indicates, elastin confers elasticity to tissues of the skin, blood vessels, lungs, bladder, and others. Elastin is a hydrolyzed protein that can be added to cosmetic products to improve skin tone and elasticity.

Glycerin

Glycerin, or glycerol, is an alcohol that can be obtained from vegetable or animal sources. Animal-sourced glycerin is a by-product of soap production that uses animal fat. Glycerin can also be a petroleum derivative. It is a humectant, which helps skin retain moisture. It is also used in the perfume industry as a solvent, as well as in many other industrial applications.

Hyaluronic acid

Hyaluronic acid, also known as hyaluronan or HA, is a natural component of the human body, mainly in the extracellular matrix. It is a major component of the vitreous humor of the eye and the synovial fluid of cartilage. It is also present in the basal layer of the epithelium at the level of the keratinocytes. Besides its numerous medical applications, HA is widely used in cosmetics as an anti-wrinkle agent, humectant, and collagen-promoting agent. Commercial HA is produced from bacteria through fermentation or isolation, or from animal sources such as synovial fluid.

Keratin

Keratin is a major protein of the skin, hair, and nails that is widely used in cosmetics, especially in hair products. Many keratin products may also contain formaldehyde, which is a highly toxic substance.

Lanolin

Lanolin is wool wax. Secreted by the sebaceous glands, it coats the wool filaments of sheep. It is a powerful skin moisturizer that provides a semi-occlusive skin barrier. It is widely used in baby products and breastfeeding nipple ointments. The United States Pharmacopeia regulates lanolin and imposes limits on its pesticide content.

Placenta extract

The placenta is a selective exchange organ that links the fetus to the mother's uterine wall. The most commonly used placenta extract is sheep placenta extract, which is used in hair products and anti-aging skin creams. Human placenta extract injections are also available as skin-rejuvenating treatments. Even though it is rich in nutrients and hormones such as estrogen and progesterone, the use of human placenta extract is associated with cultural disputes, as well as a number of restrictions and health warnings.

Squalene and Squalane

Squalene is a naturally occurring compound that is mainly obtained from shark liver oil. It can also be obtained from vegetable sources such as olives. Squalane is the hydrogenated, saturated derivative of squalene. Squalene has many applications and is sometimes used as an adjuvant in vaccines to increase immune system responsiveness. Both squalene and squalane are used as moisturizers and emollients in cosmetics.

Tallow

Tallow is usually obtained from beef fat tissues but can also come from pork and other animals. Carcasses from slaughterhouses, farms, and butchers are processed to separate fat from bone and protein. Tallow is produced through this rendering process and can be edible. It is also widely used in soap production and for animal feed.

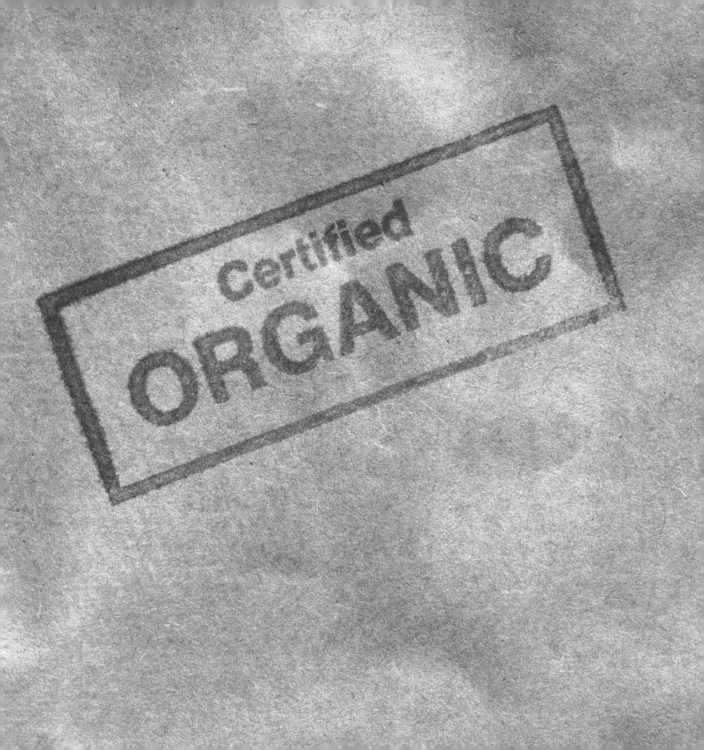

CHAPTER 19

Certifications and Seals

The increasing avoidance of questionable, mostly synthetic ingredients has started a new wave in the cosmetics industry, which has led to the birth of more natural, skin-friendly products. Many manufacturers have promised to phase out preservatives or exclude animal-derived ingredients in an attempt to satisfy consumers who do not welcome such intruders in their products.

Many other manufacturers have determined to go a step further and offer superior products that not only exclude potentially hazardous ingredients, synthetic dyes, fragrances, and petrochemicals, but also are made from strictly natural and organic ingredients.

In stores, those products are usually offered for sale in a separate section that purports to offer natural, green, and organic products, but there is no universal designation of those qualities and often poor compliance with the true definition of those terms. Ingredients within this category vary greatly, as well, which could be a source of confusion for consumers.

Because of the lack of standardization, numerous organizations have created programs that offer certification for manufacturers. A multitude of U.S., European, Canadian, and Australian organizations have been able to offer reassurance to consumers through such certification processes.

Earned seals and logos remain a credible indication of compliance with guidelines, even though those guidelines may vary greatly from one organization to another. Certification is often earned through a third party, which attests that the product has met the requirements for that specific seal. Knowing and understanding what such certifications mean can help you know and understand what you are buying and orient your choice toward more credible products.

Australian Certified Organic

The organic bud logo of Australian Certified Organic (ACO) is the most recognized organic certification in Australia, with increasing presence in the United States and Europe. ACO is a subsidiary of Australian Organic, and is the certification body and licenser of organic and biodynamic operators in Australia.

BDIH

BDIH is an international certification organization from Germany that has strict standards for the manufacture of natural cosmetics. Products that bear the BDIH certification logo may use only natural raw materials, such as plant oils, plant-derived waxes, herbal extracts, and essential oils issued from certified organic agriculture or controlled wild collection. Strict environmental guidelines are also enforced and require socially responsible production and fair trade support. All BDIH products contain natural ingredients. However, it is possible for a BDIH product to have no organic ingredients.

Biodynamic Agriculture

Biodynamic ingredients come from biodynamic agriculture, which takes things a step beyond organic. In biodynamic agriculture, plants and soil are nourished with minerals and herbs to boost their vitality; there is also respect for the plants' rhythm, influenced by astrology and other elements. It is a holistic practice that sees and respects the live interaction between plants, animals, and the solar system. Biodynamic agriculture seeks to nourish the soil instead of depleting it. Plants that are produced this way have better vitality and energy. Incorporating biodynamic ingredients is believed to nourish the skin with that vitality. Needless to say, biodynamic agriculture does not use pesticides or GMOs.

Biocosc Switzerland

For a product to obtain the Swiss Biocosc label, it must meet the following criteria: A minimum of 97 percent of the total ingredients should be natural or of natural origin; a minimum of 10 percent of the total ingredients should also come from organic agriculture; the raw natural ingredients should be obtained by simple processes and should be free of contaminants such as pesticides, GMOs, hydrocarbons, and nitrates; and the external packaging should be nonpolluting and recyclable.

The following are all strictly prohibited: parabens, phenoxyethanol, PEG, EDTA, formaldehyde, phthalates, sodium laureth sulfate, and other synthetic colorants, synthetic preservatives, synthetic fragrances, synthetic antioxidants and emollients, synthetic lipids and oils, as well as silicons and other ingredients originating from petrochemical processes, such as paraffin.

Cosmébio

Cosmébio is a French organization that, unlike Ecocert (below), does not inspect products and does not offer subsequent certification. It is simply a nonprofit organization that brings together manufacturers who intend to promote their certified organic personal care products to French and European consumers. For certification, the manufacturers must rely on another organization such as Ecocert. To be able to display the Cosmébio logo, the product must have been certified organic by a certifying agency; but not all organic-certified products will display the Cosmébio logo, unless the manufacturer chooses to become a member of Cosmébio, which remains totally optional.

Ecocert Seal

Ecocert was founded more than twenty years ago in France, where it contributed significantly to the certification of booming organic farming. Ecocert now also certifies cosmetics and perfumes, as well as paints, detergents, fertilizers, fabrics, and more. The Ecocert seal is recognized and trusted everywhere. While Ecocert Greenlife SAS handles cosmetics certification in Europe, Ecocert SA, in the United States, is accredited by the USDA under the NOP.

In 2003, Ecocert introduced the "Natural and Organic Cosmetics" standard. A cosmetics product may display the Ecocert certification logo if it meets the following criteria:

- 95 percent of the ingredients are of natural origin.

- No genetically modified ingredients exist in the finished product.

- No parabens, phenoxyethanol, petrochemicals, or synthetic chemicals are contained in the product.

- No animal testing was used in development of the product.

- The product uses recyclable or biodegradable packaging and a controlled manufacturing process.

Ecocert seems to require a low minimum of 5–10 percent organic ingredients. However, it takes into consideration all the ingredients, including salt and water. In an average product, 60 percent of the weight is water. So 10 percent of the remaining 40 percent of a product's ingredients is actually a more stringent requirement of 25 percent organic content. When the mandatory 95 percent natural ingredients requirement and the list of unacceptable ingredients are taken into consideration, Ecocert certification actually requires rigorous standards that compensate for the less than perfect organic ingredients percentage.

Fair Trade

As the name indicates, fair trade is an ethical business practice that aims at paying expected market prices for goods imported from countries with a history of exploitation. Fair Trade USA works in harmony with international standards and implements principles such as paying a guaranteed minimum floor price to democratically organized farming groups and an additional premium for certified organic products. Child labor and slavery are strictly prohibited. Safe working conditions and sustainable wages are imposed. Organizations are also offered assistance through credits (such as a pre-harvest credit) and fair trade premiums that are invested in community projects such as schooling, trainings, and organic certifications.

Fair trade encourages environment preservation through sustainable farming methods and through the prohibition of harmful agrochemicals and genetically modified organisms. Even though organic farming methods are encouraged through higher prices and special funds, not all fair trade products need to be certified organic, but they do need to be free of genetic engineering and produced with respect to the environment.

Many organizations are fair trade certifiers, such as Ecocert Fair Trade (EFT). In 2010, EFT revised its standards to better meet the global philosophy of consumers who want to purchase both eco-friendly and socially responsible products. With new standards applied to foods, textiles, and cosmetics, Ecocert Fair Trade now means both organic and fair trade.

Green

The term green is often used to mean ecofriendly, environment friendly, or earth friendly. When the definition of green is implemented through the whole production process, the resulting product will have a minimum impact on the environment. The content, the packaging, and even the manufacturing process will respect environmentally friendly procedures through the use of postconsumer recycled materials; biodegradable or recyclable packaging; sustainable, renewable ingredients that do not deplete the natural sources from which they are obtained; and green energy and energy-efficient production and manufacturing techniques that have minimal impact on the planet.

Examples of green energy include energy generated and consumed without challenging the earth's ability to handle pollution. Examples of such renewable energy technologies include hydroelectricity, wind energy, solar power, biogas, biomass, and others. The manufacturing process should also aim at minimizing energy consumption. When used efficiently, green energy resources translate into sustainable energy.

Many natural beauty products—but not all of them—are green, although green beauty products should be natural by definition. Product labeling may be required to inform the consumer that a product is ecofriendly.

NASAA Australia

NASAA is a food certification body similar to the Soil Association (p 257) that has also developed a standard for cosmetic products. NASAA limits or forbids the use of numerous synthetic ingredients and processes. Raw materials used in organic skin care products must be certified as organic, and only minimal processing is allowed in order to preserve the natural properties of the ingredients. Eco-friendly packaging material is also required. A product can be labeled "organic" only if 95 percent of its ingredients are certified organic, except for salt and water. Products can be labeled "Made with organic ingredients" if 70 percent of the ingredients (excluding salt and water) are certified organic, but such products cannot display the NASAA label.

NaTrue

The international nonprofit organization called NaTrue, from Brussels, aims at setting high standards for natural products. Members are mostly European, though the organization has an increasing international presence.

NaTrue has developed a scientific definition for natural ingredients, with different classification subcategories that make it easy to scientifically evaluate the naturalness of an ingredient:

- *Natural ingredients:* This phrase refers to those ingredients found in nature. Only physical processes may be used to obtain them; no added chemicals are allowed.

- *Derived natural substances:* These are ingredients that are found in nature but are chemically modified through a limited number of authorized processes, especially when the function of the ingredient cannot be achieved through natural ingredients. For example, surfactants in shampoos are allowed because they are essential for the cleansing function. Chemically intensive

reactions are excluded, and the surfactants must be completely biodegradable.

- *Nature-identical substances:* Nature-identical substances are substances that exist in nature but are produced synthetically for the product in question. These ingredients are permitted only in preservatives and minerals and only when the natural substance cannot be recovered from nature in the desired quality and quantity.

NaTrue offers three levels of international certification:

The first level is for products made with natural and organic ingredients, with minimal and gentle processing, as well as environmentally friendly practices. Such products do not incorporate synthetic fragrances or colors, petroleum derivatives, silicone derivatives, or genetically engineered ingredients. The irradiation of botanical ingredients or finished products is not authorized. No animal testing is allowed.

The NaTrue Natural Cosmetics seal is earned by products that meet those criteria. This level specifies which ingredients are authorized and how much processing is acceptable. There is a minimum threshold for natural ingredients and a maximum threshold for naturally derived substances for each product category.

Second level certification is met when at least 70 percent of those natural ingredients come from organic farming or wild agriculture. There is also a higher content of natural ingredients and less derived natural substances. The logo will state "Natural Cosmetics with Organic Portion."

The *third level* of certification states that the product is an "organic cosmetic" when 95 percent or more of the content is organic or wild with an even higher content of natural ingredients. Achieving this level of certification is quite a challenge for manufacturers.

No Animal Testing

Cosmetics testing on animals is particularly controversial. Such testing can involve general toxicity, eye and skin irritancy, phototoxicity, and mutagenicity. Cosmetics testing is banned in the Netherlands, Belgium, and the UK; and in 2002, after thirteen years of discussion, the European Union (EU) agreed to phase in a near-total ban on the sale of animal-tested cosmetics beginning in 2009, and to ban all cosmetics-related animal testing.

The Leaping Bunny logo indicates certification by the Coalition for Consumer Information on Cosmetics, which ensures that no new animal testing has occurred in any phase of product development by a company, its laboratories, and its ingredient suppliers. The program encourages the use of ingredients that are already known to be safe, or reliance on in vitro testing methods such as cell and tissue cultures, computer models, or even in vivo human clinical trials.

Some countries (such as China) require animal testing, and if a company in one of those countries wishes to ban animal testing for its products, it will most likely need to abandon the idea of competing in these markets.

NPA Natural Seal

Established in 1936, the Natural Products Association (formerly known as the National Nutritional Foods Association, NNFA) is the oldest and largest U.S. nonprofit organization dedicated to the natural products industry, with almost two thousand members accounting for more than ten thousand manufacturers, wholesalers, and retailers of natural products, such as health foods, sports nutrition foods, dietary supplements, and cosmetics and beauty products.

The NPA Natural Seal certification is available for personal care and home care products, as well as for ingredients. Products carrying the NPA natural seal must be made with at least 95 percent natural ingredients or naturally derived ingredients, besides water. Third-party auditors verify the amount of natural ingredients, based on certain scientific standards. The products must avoid ingredients that might pose health risks or rely on animal testing, and must also have environmentally friendly packaging. Only natural fragrances and colorants are allowed.

The Natural Products Association also offers third-party GMP (good manufacturing practices) certification, as well as yearly GMP training seminars across the United States.

Since 1997, the NPA has been hosting Natural Products Day in Washington, D.C., to interact with legislators, educate them, and seek important legislation that could have a positive impact on the natural products industry as a whole.

NSF Seal

NSF International, which identifies itself as "the public health and safety organization," is also a U.S.-based nonprofit that, along with the USDA, sets standards for cosmetics manufacturers. It also certifies water, household products, and plumbing equipment, among other things. NSF is officially recognized by the American National Standards Institute (ANSI). NSF organic standards were developed by a number of leading organic cosmetics companies. The NSF 305, the sole standard implemented by NSA International, is used to certify products that contain a minimum of 70 percent organic ingredients and are subjected to a limited number of chemical processes. Cosmetic products that meet those criteria can display the NSF "Personal Care Products Containing Organic Ingredients" on the packaging.

OASIS

OASIS stands for Organic and Sustainable Industry Standards, a nonprofit organization founded by thirty members trying to set some standards. Members are from both conventional and natural products manufacturers, with companies such as Estée Lauder and L'Oréal alongside organic lines such as Perfect Organics, Origins, and Hain Celestial (producers of Jason, Zia natural skin care, and Avalon organics).

OASIS requires a starting minimum of 85 per-cent organic content to earn the OASIS organic seal, and a 5 percent increment in organic content every couple of years until it reaches a minimum of 95 percent organic content. Otherwise, a "Made with organic" seal may be stamped on the product as long as its organic content is no less than 70 percent.

Soil Association

The Soil Association is a British organization that certifies personal care products according to two standards: For organic content of more than 95 percent (excepting water), and for organic content ranging from 70 to 95 percent. Both types may carry the Soil Association's Organic seal, but only a product with 95 percent or more organic content can include the word "organic" in the product name. Otherwise, the product may state that it is made with organic ingredients and should specify the exact percentage of organic ingredients. The seal cannot be printed on any product that contains less than 70 percent organic ingredients. The association verifies the packaging statements for accuracy before the seal is authorized.

USDA Organic Seal

In the United States, the U.S. Department of Agriculture (USDA) stands behind the National Organic Program (NOP), which defines and regulates organic agriculture.

Under NOP, the term organic is used to mean "produce or ingredients that are grown without the use of pesticides, synthetic fertilizers, sewage sludge, genetically modified organisms, or ionizing radiation."

USDA regulations that are implemented through the NOP pertain to agricultural products and foods. Because many natural products use organically grown botanical ingredients, regulations were extrapolated to include organic beauty products. The USDA organic seal can therefore be earned by a number of products made with organic ingredients.

When a beauty product is made from organic ingredients such as herbs, oils, butters, hydrosols, or essential oils, it will belong to one of four categories:

1. 100 percent organic: This refers to products made with only organic ingredients—100% of its weight (or fluid volume), except for water and salt, is made up of organic ingredients. Such a product may display the USDA organic seal.

2. Organic: This designation means that 95 percent of the ingredients (except water and salt) are organic. This product may also display the USDA organic seal.

3. Made with organic ingredients: This designation means that at least 70 percent of the ingredients (except water and salt) are organic. The main label may list up to three different ingredients, or a category of ingredients, but the product cannot display the USDA organic seal.

4. If only one or a few organic ingredients are used in the making of a product, the term organic can be used in the ingredients list but not on the principal display panel (PDP)—"the part of the

label most likely displayed or examined under customary conditions of display for sale"—and the product cannot display the USDA organic seal.

The USDA organic seal is protected by a violation fine. The USDA website states that companies who sell or label a product "organic" when they know it does not meet USDA standards can be fined up to $11,000 for each violation.

The USDA also offers a Certified Biobased Product label, which is earned by products that have a guaranteed percentage of biologically renewable ingredients from agricultural, marine, or forestry materials. The guaranteed percentage is stated on the label.

The USDA is not the only organic certification available. There are many seals that a product can carry, each representing a different certifying agency.

Vegan

There is sometimes confusion when it comes to differentiating vegan and vegetarian. While vegetarians may consume dairy products and eggs, vegans do not. Products derived from insects (such as honey, beeswax, carmine) are also often rejected by vegans. Implementing veganism can extend beyond an individual's diet when silk, leather, and other animal or insect by-products are also eliminated from clothing and furniture.

Vegan skin care products, formulated from vegetable (and synthetic) ingredients and no animal-derived products, usually say "Vegan" or "Vegan friendly" on their packaging. Honey, beeswax, and lanolin are among the ingredients that are not vegan friendly. Vegan-friendly soaps are formulated with vegetable oils and without any tallow-derived ingredients.

Cadaver tissues from both bovine and human origins are used to produce dermal fillers and other skin care ingredients that are incorporated into various anti-aging products. The main ingredient produced from such sources is collagen and collagen derivatives. Vegetable collagen does not exist, so products containing collagen or collagen derivatives are not vegan friendly.

A multitude of skin care ingredients can be obtained from either animal sources or non-animal sources; examples include stearic acid and stearates, glycerin, hyaluronic acid, and others. Referring to the supplier or manufacturer might be necessary to specify the source of the ingredient.

Substitutions Chart

The following table suggests substitutions for products that are unavailable or undesirable because of allergies or preferences. It is recommended to attempt to follow the formula, however, as it has been developed for optimum results.

SUBSTITUTE	FOR
Wheat germ, rice bran, or grape seed oil	Almond oil
Honey	Royal jelly
Glycerin	Honey
Vodka	Rubbing alcohol
Aloe vera	Cucumber juice
Flax seed	Walnuts
Grapefruit or orange	Lemon
Witch hazel	Rose water (for oily skin)
Peach or apricot kernel oil	Almond oil
Shea butter	Cocoa butter
Rice flour	Baby oatmeal or ground oats
Semolina	Almond meal

Glossary of Terms

AHA: alpha hydroxyl acids, such as glycolic acid and lactic acid, used for skin rejuvenation.

ANTIOXIDANT: a substance capable of protecting another substance from the damage caused by oxygen, such as by free radicals.

ANTISEPTIC: inhibits the growth of germs.

ASCORBIC ACID: another name for vitamin C, an essential, water-soluble vitamin found in fruits and vegetables.

ASTRINGENT: a substance capable of constricting body tissues, reducing bleeding and secretions; cosmetic applications of astringent substances help reduce the size of skin pores.

BETA-CAROTENE: belongs to the group of carotenoids, which are antioxidants converted to vitamin A.

BIODYNAMIC: an ecological, spiritual, and ethical approach to agriculture and nutrition.

COMEDOGENIC: capable of clogging pores, leading to the formation of blackheads.

DIURETIC: a substance that encourages urine formation and loss of retained water.

EMOLLIENT: a substance capable of softening and soothing skin.

EMULSIFIER: a substance that is added to a liquid to promote the cohesion of oil and water.

ENZYMES: proteins produced by living organisms that are capable of inducing chemical reactions and transforming substrates.

EPIDERMIS: the most exterior, nonvascular layer of skin.

ESSENTIAL FATTY ACIDS: unsaturated fatty acids, which are essential for bodily functions and cannot be synthetized by the human body.

EXFOLIATION: the act of exfoliating, which consists of scaling off or peeling off dead skin cells at the surface of the epidermis.

FAIR TRADE: an ethical business practice that aims at paying expected market prices for goods imported from countries with a history of exploitation.

GERMICIDAL: actively killing germs (not only prohibiting their growth).

GREEN: ecofriendly, environment friendly, or earth friendly; used to describe products that have minimum impact on the environment.

HUMECTANT: a substance that helps retain moisture.

HYDROSOL: herbal or flower water, also known as an herbal distillate, obtained by the steam distillation of herbs or flowers.

KERATOLYTIC: a substance capable of inducing the softening and shedding of the skin's thick keratin layers; often used for wart removal.

MICROCIRCULATION: circulation of blood through the fine vessels.

MICRONUTRIENTS: nutrients needed in very tiny amounts to maintain physiological functions.

MOISTURIZER: a cosmetic cream or lotion used to hydrate the upper layers of the epidermis and counteract dry skin.

OMEGA-3: a type of essential fatty acid that is abundant in fish oils and can provide multiple health benefits such as lowering LDL cholesterol and raising HDL cholesterol.

OMEGA-6: a type of essential fatty acid abundant in vegetable oils, eggs, and meats; the dietary intake of omega-6 versus omega-3 fatty acids is often exceedingly elevated.

ORGANIC: "produce or ingredients that are grown without the use of pesticides, synthetic fertilizers, sewage sludge, genetically modified organisms, or ionizing radiation" (from the NOP).

OXIDATION: a chemical reaction of oxygen resulting in loss of electrons in the original substance; oxidation is considered to be a deterioration of oils.

PANTOTHENIC ACID: also known as vitamin B5, this water-soluble vitamin is widely present in food and has antioxidant properties.

PHOTOSENSITIVITY: an increased sensitivity to light and UV radiation.

PUFA: polyunsaturated fatty acids; fatty acids that have more than one unsaturated double or triple bond in their molecules.

RANCIDITY: the state of an oil or fat that has undergone oxidation; implies an unpleasant smell and taste.

SEBUM: oily secretion produced by the sebaceous skin glands to lubricate the skin.

SURFACTANT: compoud that lowers surface tension between two liquids or between a liquid and a solid.

TANNINS: antioxidative phenolic compounds found in plants, tea, and wine, capable of precipitating proteins.

THICKENER: a substance that is capable of increasing the viscosity of a product.

TOCOPHEROLS: a group of closely related fat-soluble compounds that form vitamin E.

VEGAN: free from animal products and by-products; vegans avoid eating or using animal-derived foods and goods.

VOLATILE: evaporates easily and rapidly.

Disclaimer

The information contained in this book is for practical guidance purposes only.

The author has carefully constructed all formulas listed in this book, a selection based on scientific knowledge, relevant trainings, professional experience, and available information.

The author is not accountable for unforeseen consequences, allergic reactions, dissatisfying results, or misinterpretation or misuse of the formulas. The author's opinions and suggestions should not replace a physician's advice.

The content of this book has not been evaluated by the FDA and is not intended to diagnose, treat, or cure any disease, including dermatological conditions. Please consult with your physician first.

In very rare instances, some ingredients (such as grapefruit) may interact with medication you might be taking. Please consult with your physician prior to using such formulas.

Supplement at your own risk. Any vitamins, minerals, or other supplements inspired by the content of this book should be approved by a physician.

People with special medical conditions, pregnant women, breastfeeding women, elderly people, children, and people on medication should consult with their physician before using formulas from this book.

Some formulas might call for allergens such as nuts, nut oils, dairy, or eggs. Do not use in cases of a known allergy, and always perform a patch test prior to applying.

Besides the formulas that are especially mentioned as suitable for irritated skin, do not use any formula on irritated skin or open wounds.

People with asthma, COPD, or other respiratory conditions should consult with your physician prior to working with essential oils, powders, or alcohols.

Acknowledgments

With very sincere gratitude for every contributor to the concretization of "Natural Beauty Alchemy":

My agent, Coleen O'Shea of the Allen O'Shea Literary agency, who saw beyond my dreams and guided me through every step of the way, little or big, with professional commitment and efficiency.

The Countryman Press staff, especially editors Ann Treistman and Sarah Bennett, who worked diligently and attentively to create a book beyond expectations.

Wael Hamza, from F&J House production, whose photographs captured the art of natural beauty and poured it on colored page.

I hope this book is all what you expect and so much more.

THANK YOU!

INDEX

Photo Credits